Get the

TRANS FAT

Out

Get the
TRANS FAT
Out

601 Simple Ways

to Cut the Trans Fat

Out of Any Diet

Suzanne Havala Hobbs

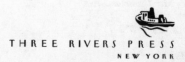

THREE RIVERS PRESS
NEW YORK

Copyright © 2006 by Suzanne Havala Hobbs

All rights reserved.
Published in the United States by Three Rivers Press, an imprint of the Crown Publishing Group, a division of Random House, Inc., New York.
www.crownpublishing.com

Three Rivers Press and the Tugboat design are registered trademarks of Random House, Inc.

For a complete listing of credits, see page 274.

Library of Congress Cataloging-in-Publication Data

Hobbs, Suzanne Havala.
Get the trans fat out : 601 simple ways to cut the trans fat out of any diet /
Suzanne Havala Hobbs.—1st ed.
p.   cm.
Includes index.
1. Low-fat diet. 2. Trans fatty acids. 3. Lipids in human nutrition.
4. Low-fat diet—Recipes. I. Title.
RM237.7.H63 2006
613.2'84—dc22

ISBN-13: 978-0-307-34198-3
ISBN-10: 0-307-34198-4

Printed in the United States of America

Design by Meryl Sussman Levavi

10 9 8 7 6 5 4 3 2 1

First Edition

To the readers of my newspaper column, "On the Table," and people everywhere in search of sound, practical advice about how best to eat to support health

Contents

"A loaf of bread," the Walrus said,
"is what we chiefly need:
Pepper and vinegar besides
Are very good indeed."

—LEWIS CARROLL,
Through the Looking Glass

Preface

Trans fat is what happens when food manufacturers add hydrogen to vegetable oil, and it is very bad for you. It contributes to obesity, and even the slightest amount in your diet raises your risk of heart disease, according to a major report by the Institute of Medicine. Eating trans fat is worse for your health than eating lard.

The problem: Trans fat is everywhere. It's in cakes, cookies, pies, muffins, fast-food french fries and sandwiches, frozen entrees, salad dressings, margarine, and more. And it's elusive. Nutrition information isn't posted on the labels of fast-food products, and until recently, food packagers didn't have to reveal the amount of trans fat in their products on the food's label. Clues on ingredient labels—the presence of partially hydrogenated vegetable oils, for example—have long been the only practical means of learning whether a product contains harmful trans fat. Until now.

In January 2006, the federal government put into effect new regulations requiring food manufacturers to list on the food labels the amount of trans fat contained in their products. This change has set into motion a flurry of new trans-fat-free product development and the reformulation of other products.

But the world won't be rid of trans fat anytime soon. Trans fat is ubiquitous because the food industry hasn't yet found an economical substitute that functions the same way. Fast-food companies will continue to use trans fat, and while the new labeling law will make trans fat easier to find in packaged foods, most of us will still need help understanding how best to dodge it, which products are okay to eat, and how to adopt and maintain a trans-fat-free lifestyle. This book provides this information along with a quick reference fat counter that puts the newly available trans fat content of popular products at your fingertips.

In this book you'll find

- an explanation of what trans fat is, how it came to be, and how it affects your health.
- advice on how to choose foods free of trans fat.
- a complete, up-to-date fat counter listing the grams of trans fat and saturated fat in a comprehensive range of food products.
- brand-specific and generic food information to help you get started.
- most important, advice that puts health and nutrition information into perspective, highlighting the most pertinent facts and explaining what they mean in terms of shopping, preparing meals, and choosing foods away from home.

The biggest challenge most of us face is *how* to eat well. My aim in this book is to give you the information and tools you need to help yourself eat well and stay healthy. Getting the trans fat out is one vital step.

Introduction

This book will give you the basic information about trans fat: what it is, how it affects your health, and how to cut it out of your diet by choosing the right foods and planning healthy meals. When you have finished reading this book, you should be armed with knowledge and practical advice that you can put to use right away.

How to Use This Book

What information do you need to understand how to eat a diet free of trans fat? How do you prefer to learn it? Your answers to these questions will determine how you should use this book. Do what works for you. Here are some options for how to use it.

◆ *Read it from cover to cover.* Reading it all will give you a comprehensive understanding of the issues. Understanding the background—what trans fat is and how it affects your health—will help put into perspective the advice on planning meals that exclude it. A solid overview of the topic will equip you to make good decisions when you're faced with food choices.

♦ *Go surfing.* Some people can't sit still long enough to read a self-help book from cover to cover (I count myself among them). We'd rather jump around, read a little here and there, and pick up ideas and inspiration along the way. That's fine, but at the very least I recommend that you read the first section of Chapter 1 on what trans fat is, the section of Chapter 2 on the health effects of trans fat, and the sections of Chapter 3 that discuss how to read nutrition facts labels on foods and how to make sense of ingredient labels. You'll then have the fundamentals, and you can flip through the tips in the rest of the book to gain ideas and inspiration where you need them.

♦ *Troubleshoot with it.* If you don't have the time to read the book now, keep it handy and use it as a reference. As you read food labels and run into snags, return to the book for a primer on label reading. If a question about the function of trans fat in foods pops into your head, go to the book for the answer. You can also use the food counter in Part III to find out quickly if your favorite foods are sources of trans fat and then identify substitutes if you need them.

The book is meant to be a practical tool to help you learn the basics and make the best decisions about what to feed yourself and your family. The focus is trans fat, but the advice given also steers you toward choices that support overall health.

How This Book Is Organized

The book is divided into three parts.

Part I: A Trans Fat Primer offers basic scientific and health information.

♦ Chapter 1: Understanding Trans Fat explains what trans

fat is, how it came to be, why food companies like to use it, and where it is found.

◆ Chapter 2: Trans Fat and Your Health examines the health effects of trans fat—why it is worse for you than lard—as well as how trans fat compares with other types of fats. This chapter covers dietary recommendations for trans fat, including an important report issued by the Institute of Medicine and a discussion of setting personal goals for intakes of trans fat.

◆ Chapter 3: Regulations and Label Logic explains the new regulations for listing the trans fat content of foods on product labels. Sample food labels are included along with instructions for reading and interpreting the nutrition facts information and ingredient lists. You'll also learn what to do when foods don't come with a label.

◆ Chapter 4: Putting It All Together puts information about trans fat into perspective and discusses the issue in the context of your total diet. Included is advice on crafting an approach to dealing with trans fat that works with your lifestyle, where to get additional help if you need it, and tips on how to get started on eliminating trans fat from your diet.

Part II: Getting the Trans Fat Out gets to the nitty-gritty of putting dietary advice about trans fat into practice. Nine chapters provide detailed advice and a wide range of practical tips for getting the trans fat out of all the foods you eat at home and away. You'll discover how to get the trans fat out of your pantry and refrigerator and what to look out for in breads, salad dressings and dips, entrees and side dishes, snacks, baked goods, desserts, and treats—whether you're eating at home or at a restaurant.

Part III: The Food Guide and Fat Gram Counter contains a handy reference guide that lists the trans fat, saturated fat, and combined trans fat and saturated fat ("bad fat") contents of more than 1,500 foods in the supermarket and restaurants.

You can use the food guide and fat gram counter in a few different ways:

◆ To construct a shopping list. Use the guide to identify trans-fat-free foods and foods in various categories that are low in bad fats.

◆ To lobby for more choices in stores. If you see trans-fat-free products listed that your local supermarket doesn't stock but you'd like to buy, bring this to the attention of your store manager. Store managers will often stock an item if they think others will buy it, too. In other cases, a store may require that you buy an entire carton or case of that product.

◆ To check the trans fat content of your favorite foods. Use the guide to find out whether the foods you eat most often are sources of trans fat. If a favorite food contains trans fat, you can use the guide to find a trans-fat-free substitute.

Use this book to guide yourself to a healthier diet.

Please Note: The information contained in this book is general and is not intended as personal medical advice for an individual's specific health problems. If you are seriously ill or on medication, please check with your medical doctor or health care provider before changing your diet.

PART I

A Trans Fat Primer

The first part of this book is devoted to explaining why it's important to get the trans fat out of your diet. It is the background you need to help you put the issue into perspective as well as help you make informed decisions when making food choices. As you read this part of the book, think about the foods you eat today that are high in trans fat—those you keep in your kitchen as well as those you eat when you're at a restaurant. Once you're aware of where trans fat hides in your diet and why you need to get it out, the remainder of this book will help you accomplish that goal.

Chapter 1

Understanding Trans Fat

For many years you had to know what you were looking for to find any clue that your favorite foods might contain trans fat. That's because the government didn't require food manufacturers to list trans fat on product nutrition labels, and so almost universally they did not list it.

The effect was that most of us paid no attention to how much trans fat we were eating even though partially hydrogenated oils—the main source of trans fat—were being used in 40 percent of the foods sold in supermarkets. But people are paying attention now.

Science has found serious health risks associated with eating partially hydrogenated oils and other sources of trans fat. Trans fat is dangerous because it raises blood levels of LDL, or "bad" cholesterol, while also lowering levels of HDL, or "good" cholesterol.

How bad is that? A large study that examined, among other things, links between diet and health—The Nurses Health Study—has shown that women who eat twice the average amount of trans fat (about 5 grams or 1 teaspoon per day) developed 62 percent more heart disease than the average. Other studies have provided preliminary evidence that trans fat causes general inflammation in the body, an emerging risk factor for coronary artery disease, heart failure, diabetes, and other conditions.

Health professionals are therefore advising us to severely limit or eliminate trans fat from our diets. For the first time new federal regulations are requiring food manufacturers to list the trans fat content of their products on food labels. In response to these new rules, many companies are reformulating their products to reduce or rid them of trans fat.

Let me be clear: Trans fats are very bad for you. They cause many health problems, and they contribute to obesity. You do need some fat, but trans fat is a bad fat that should be eliminated from your diet and replaced with good fats.

Trans fat won't disappear overnight. It will be years before we see the end of partially hydrogenated oils in packaged and manufactured foods. It will be necessary for you to make some changes to cut trans fat out of your diet.

You need to understand some basics before you begin: what hydrogenated oils and other sources of trans fat are, where they come from, why they are used, and where they are found.

What Are Trans Fats?

Our bodies store fat so that it can be burned later for energy, the energy needed to fuel the work our bodies perform as they grow and develop. Fats, also called fatty acids, serve a variety of other functions, such as helping to transport fat-soluble vitamins A, D, E, and K throughout the body. We need some fat to be healthy, but most of us get too much of the wrong kinds from the foods we eat.

There are three main forms of fat in our diets: monounsaturated fat, polyunsaturated fat, and saturated fat. Each has a unique chemical configuration and functions differently in the body.

Most fats occur naturally in foods. Trans fat is a somewhat different case. Some trans fats occur naturally in dairy products and meats. Most, however, are man-made. Trans fat is created when vegetable oil is put through a process called hydrogenation. In this process, hydrogen gas is bubbled through liquid vegetable oil, causing a change in the chemical configuration of the oil and making it thicker in consistency.

Oil can be hydrogenated a little or a lot. Hydrogenate just a little, as in partially hydrogenated oils, and you get an oil substance with the consistency of soft margarine. More hydrogenation creates a more solid product, such as canned shortenings.

When food manufacturers fully hydrogenate oil, they create a product that no longer contains trans fat. But fully hydrogenated oils are very hard and waxlike. They have limited use in foods unless combined with other oils—such as liquid sunflower oil and soy oils—to create a softer consistency. On the other hand, partially hydrogenated oils—known as "plastic fats" in the food business—have special properties that make them invaluable to food manufacturers, especially in baking. Among other things, plastic fats help create flakier piecrusts and biscuits and extend the shelf lives of processed foods.

A Little Bit of Trans Fat History

The process of using hydrogen gas to convert liquid oil to solid fat was pioneered in Germany and England more than one hundred years ago, but it was Procter & Gamble that brought partially hydrogenated oils to the masses. It came in millions of cans labeled with the name Crisco.

A Comparison of the Chemical Configuration of Fats

A saturated fat has a chemical structure that looks like this:

Saturated Fat

H H
||
-C-C-
||
H H

**Carbon-Carbon
Single Bond**

An unsaturated fat has a chemical structure that looks like this:

Unsaturated Fat

H H
||
-C=C-

**Carbon-Carbon
Double Bond**

A trans fat has a chemical structure that looks like this:

Trans Fat

H
|
-C=C-
|
H

**Hydrogen atoms are on opposite sides of the chain of
carbon atoms at the carbon-carbon double bond.**

Source: U.S. Food and Drug Administration, Center for Food Safety and Applied Nutrition

As the twentieth century began, P&G needed to come up with new products. Electricity was spreading across the land, massively cutting demand for the firm's candles. Meatpackers were cornering the market on lard, another of P&G's main products. The company would be in major trouble if it didn't come up with new innovations to sell to American households.

In 1907, a German chemist named E. C. Kayser wrote to company officials asking whether they would be interested in his discoveries in the field of hydrogenation. The company had recently made progress in research on processing cottonseed oil so that it could remain liquid in cold temperatures, but P&G researchers were having trouble creating a solid form of the oil—one that could compete with lard, butter, and other cooking products.

Kayser accepted the company's invitation to the firm's headquarters in Cincinnati and, according to company lore, showed up with a white block that he placed on the desk of P&G chief Cooper Procter.

"What's that?" Procter asked.

"Cottonseed oil," Kayser replied.

P&G quickly hired Kayser, and by 1911 the company had perfected the production of what would come to be known as Crisco, a creamy white shortening suitable for use in cakes and pastries and with properties similar to lard but less likely to become rancid. It had the added advantage of being cheaper than butter, and it could be produced and used in baked goods with consistent results.

The first advertisement for Crisco appeared in the *Ladies' Home Journal* in 1912, declaring it to be "an absolutely new product. A scientific discovery which will affect every kitchen in America." And it did.

P&G established traveling "cooking schools" that hosted demonstrations nationwide to teach American housewives how to cook with Crisco. Free recipes and inexpensive cookbooks were distributed to housewives. By 1921, Crisco ads asked, "Why have a smoky kitchen?" and promised women they would be "out of the kitchen by noon!" In 1931, housewives across the country tuned in to a regular radio program called *Mrs. Blake's Radio Column.* Twice a week the program featured a Sisters of the Skillet cooking segment that promoted the use of Crisco shortening.

Another Crisco advertisement from the early 1930s showed

a motherly "Mrs. Paul" entering a distraught woman's kitchen holding a can of Crisco; she was there to show the woman how to make "a light and digestible pie that will delight her husband's boss when he comes to dinner."

It didn't take long for Crisco to revolutionize home baking by becoming the best-selling all-purpose household vegetable shortening in the United States.

Why Food Companies Love Trans Fat

Crisco and other partially hydrogenated oils helped alter the way homemakers baked and completely changed the American diet.

Partially hydrogenated oils came onto the food scene just as the country—indeed, the world—entered the era of mass production of consumer products. Automobiles, washing machines, sewing machines, refrigerators, and other consumer goods became more common as industrialization took hold. Hand in hand with the growing availability of time-saving appliances came changes in modern life as more households found their breadwinners rushing from home in the morning to go to factory jobs.

Convenience became a selling point for many products, including food. Widening use of partially hydrogenated oils meant that foods such as cakes, pies, cookies, and doughnuts could be made in factories and shipped to grocery stores. "Store-bought" cakes set the new standard for baking quality.

The food industry began widely adopting the use of partially hydrogenated oils. Cost was one factor. Partially hydrogenated vegetable oils could take the place of—and cost less than—butter and lard in most foods. Better still, hydrogenated oils increased the shelf life of foods, because they went rancid much more slowly than butter and lard.

Hydrogenated oils are useful in other ways, too. They make

crackers and cookies crisp, keep cakes moist, and add a good flavor to foods. They don't break down as quickly as liquid oils, so fast-food companies and other restaurants can use them longer in deep-fat fryers for cooking French fries, fried pies, chicken nuggets, breaded fish, and other foods.

A century after trans fat was introduced into the American diet, fully 40 percent of the products sold in grocery stores contained it. Use of hydrogenated oil is so widespread in the food industry that removing it—or substantially lowering dependence on its use—presents a major challenge. Not only do substitutes for hydrogenated oils cost more, but they also taste different. Part of the challenge for the food industry in finding ways to remove trans fat is creating new recipes that closely match the familiar flavors and textures of popular foods.

In some cases, the food industry has succeeded. Just as Crisco ushered in the era of trans fat, the baking staple recently underwent another transformation as attention shifted to the dangers of trans fat. The shortening, which is now owned by J. M. Smucker Co., has been reformulated with a blend of sunflower, soy, and cottonseed oils to remove trans fat. The new version of the old staple is called "Crisco 0 Grams Trans Fat Shortening."

But many of our favorite foods still contain trans fat. It's up to you to find them and cut them out of your diet.

Where to Find Them

The lists below contain many but not all of the most common sources of trans fat in foods. Remember, at last count, trans fat was being used in more than forty thousand products on supermarket shelves. In Chapter 3 you will learn how to read food labels so that you can check for the presence of trans fat in foods and avoid them.

Food manufacturers are working to remove trans fat from many products, but other foods will still contain trans fat, because it may take years before some products can be reformulated. And since restaurants aren't required to disclose the trans fat content of menu items, you'll need to continue to be careful when you eat out as well.

Of course, some foods never contained trans fat at all. Foods that are not processed and are close to their natural state don't have trans fat. They're given in the lists, along with foods that contain naturally occurring trans fat. It's not yet known whether naturally occurring trans fats confer the same health risks as those that are man-made. However, the foods that contain trans fat—cheese, whole milk, and meat, for example—are also rich sources of artery-clogging saturated fat, so avoiding them is a good idea regardless of the health risks of the trans fat.

TRANS FAT IN FOODS: WHERE TO FIND IT

FOODS THAT NEVER CONTAIN TRANS FAT

FRESH FRUITS: apples, bananas, blueberries, cherries, cantaloupe, grapes, kiwi, mangoes, papayas, peaches, pineapple, watermelon, and others

FRESH VEGETABLES: asparagus, broccoli, cauliflower, celery, green beans, onions, potatoes, sweet potatoes, tomatoes, winter squash, zucchini, and others

LEGUMES: black beans, garbanzo beans, kidney beans, navy beans, pinto beans, lentils, split peas, and others

PLAIN GRAINS: barley, old-fashioned rolled oats, whole wheat hot cereal, white and brown rice, and others

FOODS THAT CONTAIN TRANS FAT NATURALLY

MEATS: beef, lamb, pork

DAIRY PRODUCTS: butter, cheese, ice cream, milk, sour cream, whipping cream, yogurt, and others

FOODS WITH ADDED TRANS FAT

These foods are the leading sources of harmful trans fat. You should avoid them to protect your health.

Cake and brownie mixes

Commercial baked goods: cakes, cookies, biscuits, pastries, and pies

Crackers

Homemade baked goods made with solid shortening (butter, regular margarine, or regular Crisco-type solid shortening)

Fast food: French fries, fried chicken, fish, pies, and other deep-fried foods

Frozen entrees

Frozen waffles

Ready-to-eat frosting

Margarine

Microwave popcorn

Solid vegetable shortening such as Crisco

Restaurant foods: Deep-fried foods, commercial baked goods, grilled sandwiches made with butter or margarine, and others

Part III of this book contains a food guide and fat gram counter that lists the trans fat and saturated fat content of more than 1,500 brand-name and generic foods.

Chapter 2

Trans Fats and Your Health

Have you ever heard the saying, "I've read so much about the dangers of eating that I've decided to give up reading"?

It's not hard to understand the frustration. Advice about diet and health often appears contradictory, confusing, or simply too difficult to follow. In the case of trans fats, putting advice into practice is a challenge because trans fats are in so many of the foods we eat. Until now, trans fats in foods were largely hidden, since their presence wasn't recorded on the nutrition facts label on products. Even now, with mandatory reporting of trans fats on food labels, trans fats are still hidden in many foods that don't come with labels, such as foods sold in restaurants and bakeries.

In the next chapter we'll tackle making sense of label information about trans fats and what to do if the information isn't there. Before we get to that, though, it's important to understand the nature of trans fats and why you should care.

This chapter lays out the scientific links between trans fats and your health and explains what matters and what doesn't. We'll cover how trans fats affect health, how trans fats compare to other kinds of fat in your diet, what health authorities recommend you do about including or excluding trans fats in your diet, and precisely how to approach your personal dietary goals.

Health Effects of Trans Fats (or Why Trans Fats Are as Bad for Your Health as Lard)

Dietary recommendations about trans fats stem from associations between trans fats and the risk factors for coronary artery disease as well as the incidence of heart disease itself.

Throughout the 1980s and 1990s, preliminary research findings on trans fats suggested that trans fats either had no negative effects on health or they raised cholesterol levels, though not as much as did the saturated fats in meat, cheese, and other animal products. For that reason many health advocates urged the use and consumption of trans fats in food products. That's why margarine was once thought to be better for you than butter.

But—as is often the case in nutritional research—the science related to trans fats has evolved significantly. A much larger body of evidence from the most rigorous types of studies has accumulated, reversing earlier findings and offering stronger evidence that trans fats raise the risk of coronary artery disease. Today there is scientific consensus that trans fats pose a serious risk to health. The evidence shows that foods containing trans fats raise the body's level of the most dangerous form of blood cholesterol: LDL, or low-density lipoprotein. At the same time trans fats lower a protective form of blood cholesterol: HDL, or high-density lipoprotein, sometimes referred to as "good cholesterol." High-density lipoproteins help remove dangerous forms of cholesterol from the body. You want blood levels of HDL to be relatively high and LDL levels to be low. Foods that contain trans fats have the opposite effect.

The case against trans fats doesn't stop there. Epidemiological studies, which follow the diet and disease patterns of groups of people, have also found that the more trans fat people eat, the higher their rates of coronary artery disease. The evidence that trans fats harm health is so strong that the Food and Drug Administration concluded in 2003: "Because of the serious public health consequences of CHD [coronary heart disease] in the U.S. population, prudent public health dictates that we help consumers control those risk factors which they can alter directly through their own behavior. Heart healthy diets that limit the intakes of both saturated and trans fats can serve this purpose as is evidenced by recommendations in the recent expert panel reports."

How Trans Fats Compare with Other Fats

All fats do not have the same health risks. Some are better or worse for health than others.

Before trans fats were found to pose health risks, most dietary advice emphasized the need for lower intakes of saturated fat and cholesterol. Here is a brief tutorial on what these terms mean and how different types of fats compare:

Cholesterol

Cholesterol actually isn't a fat at all. Instead, it's a waxlike substance produced in the liver. We need cholesterol for the production of hormones, cell membranes, and vitamin D, but our bodies produce all we need.

Some people are genetically predisposed to produce too much cholesterol. For others, what they eat may cause their bodies to produce more cholesterol than they need. People can also get excessive amounts of cholesterol from foods. However it happens, when blood cholesterol levels are elevated, the excess can contribute to a buildup of plaque in the arteries. That can cause narrowing of the arteries and coronary artery disease.

Cholesterol is found in all animal products, including meat, eggs, and cheese, and there is no cholesterol in any foods that come from the soil. Saturated fat and trans fat in the diet can also cause the liver to produce more cholesterol.

Saturated Fat

Saturated fat and trans fat are two different things, but they both raise blood cholesterol levels.

Saturated fat is generally solid at room temperature. Think of a block of butter or a tub of lard. Saturated fats are found in animal products such as milk, sour cream, ice cream, yogurt, cheese, meat, and poultry.

Most of the saturated fat in the American diet comes from dairy products, and about two-thirds of the fat in dairy products is in the saturated form. Do you like pizza and grilled cheese sandwiches? How much ice cream do you eat, and how often do you add sour cream to a baked potato or a plate of nachos? Foods such as these provide most of the saturated fat in our diets. According to expert panels that helped develop federal dietary guidelines and recommendations, an average of 11 percent to 12 percent of the calories we consume each day come from saturated fats. In comparison, trans fats contribute about 3 percent of calories in our diets each day.

Tropical oils—for example, coconut oil, cocoa butter, and palm oil—also contain saturated fats. Tropical oils are used in candies, cookies, cakes, and other commercial baked goods. Some nuts also contain small amounts of saturated fat.

Saturated fats act much like trans fats in the body: They increase the body's production of LDL cholesterol and with it the risk for coronary artery disease. Some researchers have

questioned whether trans fats have an effect on LDL cholesterol levels that is less than, equal to, or greater than that of saturated fats. According to the Food and Drug Administration's
assessment of the research, it's not possible to know the answer
given the evidence available at this time, but the effects are
likely similar.

Unsaturated Fats

Other forms of fat don't pose the health risks that saturated fats
and trans fats do. In fact, some fats are beneficial to health and
can lower blood cholesterol levels.

Unsaturated fats are sometimes called "good fats" because
they can raise the levels of HDL (the "good" cholesterol) and
lower the levels of LDL (the "bad" cholesterol). Unsaturated fats
are found in plant foods such as vegetable oils, nuts, and seeds.

There are two primary forms of unsaturated fats: monounsaturated and polyunsaturated. They have different chemical
configurations, but both are beneficial to health. Examples of
foods rich in monounsaturated fat include canola, peanut, and
olive oils. Sunflower, corn, and soybean oils are rich in polyunsaturated fat. To protect your health, aim for replacing saturated
and trans fats with polyunsaturated and monounsaturated fats.

The table below summarizes the primary types of dietary
fats and their sources and effects on health.

TYPE OF FAT	SOURCES	HEALTH EFFECTS
Trans	Regular margarines; solid vegetable shortening; partially hydrogenated vegetable oils; fast-food French fries and other deep-fried foods; com-mercial baked goods and other foods	Raises LDL and lowers HDL, increasing the risk of coronary artery disease

TYPE OF FAT	SOURCES	HEALTH EFFECTS
Saturated	Whole milk, cheese, butter, sour cream, yogurt, ice cream, meat, cocoa butter, coconut oil, and palm oil	Raises LDL and HDL, and increases the risk of coronary artery disease
Polyunsaturated	Corn, soybean, safflower, and cottonseed oils, and fish.	Lowers LDL, raises HDL, and reduces the risk of coronary artery disease
Monounsaturated	Olives, avocados, nuts, nut butters, olive oil, canola oil, and peanut oil	Lowers LDL, raises HDL, and reduces the risk of coronary artery disease

Dietary Recommendations for Trans Fats: How Much Is Too Much?

Government dietary advice on trans fats is concerned with what is best as well as what is practical.

Recent major scientific reports on trans fats all conclude the same thing: Intakes of trans fats should be kept as low as possible. Reports issued by expert committees for the Dietary Guidelines for Americans, the National Cholesterol Education Program, and the Institute of Medicine advise that intakes of saturated fat and trans fat should be kept as low as possible to reduce the risk of coronary artery disease in the general population as well as for those at high risk for heart disease.

In its report, the Institute of Medicine stated that even small amounts of trans fat in the diet were associated with an increased risk of coronary artery disease. In fact, if a "tolerable upper intake level" were to be set, it would be zero. In other words, there is no safe level of intake of trans fat.

The researchers who drafted the IOM report felt, however, that it would be unrealistic to tell Americans to eat zero trans fats. Trans fats are so widespread in the American food supply that most people would probably be unable to avoid them completely without making extraordinary changes in their diets. Doing so could cause people to so restrict their diets that they would end up eating insufficient amounts of other needed nutrients. Instead, the final report recommended that "trans fat consumption be as low as possible while consuming a nutritionally adequate diet."

So if the ultimate goal is really zero but getting to zero would be difficult, what is a realistic goal for your intake of trans fat? A practical approach is to lump trans fat with saturated fat and follow guidelines for the intake of saturated fat to determine a reasonable intake level.

Similar to trans fats, the IOM also concluded that there is no safe level of intake of saturated fat; however, a longstanding recommendation for the intake of saturated fat has set the limit at not more than 10 percent of total calories. The final figure—the number of combined grams of saturated and trans fat that you should limit yourself to each day—varies depending on how many calories you need as well as the percentage of calories from fat that your diet contains.

For example, if your diet contains 2,000 calories per day, and you limit your fat intake to 30 percent of the calories, 600 calories each day should come from fat. Here is the math: 2,000 x 0.30 = 600. There are 9 calories in a gram of fat, so that means your total fat intake should be no more than about 67 grams. Here's the math: 600 ÷ 9 = 66.6.

Less than 10 percent of the calories in your diet should come from saturated fat. Using the same example, then, less than 200 calories should come from saturated fat. Here's the math: 2,000 x 0.10 = 200. Divide 200 calories by 9 calories in a gram of fat, and you get 22. So, of the 67 grams of fat in your diet, no more than about 20 grams should come from saturated fat.

Of course, now we're saying that figure, 20 grams of fat, should represent the *combined* limit of saturated fat and trans fat. (You should also keep your intake of cholesterol as low as possible.) Lower than that is even better.

Also consider that 2,000 calories is a relatively high calorie intake. Many people, including those who need to lose weight, should eat fewer calories than that.

Let's say that your calorie needs are about 1,500 per day, which is typical for most women and many men who are trying to lose weight. Given that calorie intake, the combined limit for saturated and trans fat intakes would be about 16 grams per day. Again, lower is even better.

The next chapter will show you how to use new information on food labels to help you meet your goals.

Chapter 3

Regulations and Label Logic

Trans fat labeling has been a long time coming. Saturated fat and cholesterol have been required to be listed on food labels since 1993. In 1994, the Center for Science in the Public Interest, a consumer advocacy organization, petitioned the Food and Drug Administration—the federal agency that oversees labeling regulations for foods and nutritional supplements—to require food manufacturers to include trans fat on food labels.

According to CSPI, a substantial body of scientific evidence had accumulated showing that dietary trans fats raised blood cholesterol levels, increasing the risk of coronary artery disease. The group claimed that then-current regulations did not adequately reflect the effect of dietary trans fatty acids on the risk for heart disease and that label values for saturated fat underestimated the total amount of "heart-unhealthy" fats if trans fats were not also listed.

In response, the FDA in 1999 started the formal process for making a regulatory change to add trans fat to nutrition facts labels by publishing a proposed rule in the *Federal Register*. The proposal was open to public comment and underwent several revisions before it was finalized in 2003. Among the more controversial changes proposed by the FDA was the inclusion of a nutrition label footnote that read: "Intake of trans fat should be as low as possible." The food industry resisted the addition of the statement, saying that it represented dietary advice and that food labels should state data only. The footnote requirement was removed from the final rule.

The final rule took into consideration comments from scientists, food companies and other industry representatives, citizens, health professionals, and others who had stakes in trans fats being listed on food labels. Since political and economic issues, in addition to science, factored into the deliberations, the new rule isn't ideal in terms of how health information about trans fats is conveyed on nutrition labels. It is a good start, though, and the new regulation does ensure that consumers have access to the most vital information—the trans fat content of foods—which is needed to make careful, informed decisions about what to buy and eat.

In this chapter we'll look at what food labels say about trans fat and what they leave out. We'll cover how to read and interpret nutrition facts labels, how to make sense of ingredient lists, and what to do when the information isn't there.

What Labels Say About Trans Fats, and What They Don't

Look at the sample food label below. Find where trans fat is listed under the heading for total fat.

Trans fat is listed on the nutrition facts label on a separate line beneath the heading of total fat. Saturated fat is also listed on a separate line. You'll notice in the example that in this product the total of saturated fat and trans fat together add up to less than the total fat per serving in the product. The difference can be accounted for by the amount of unsaturated fat in the product, which is not listed.

Nutrition Facts

Serving Size 1 cup (228g)
Servings Per Container 2

Amount Per Serving

Calories 260   Calories from Fat 120

	% Daily Value*
Total Fat 13g	**20%**
Saturated Fat 5g	**25%**
Trans Fat 2g	
Cholesterol 30mg	**10%**
Sodium 660mg	**28%**
Total Carbohydrate 31g	**10%**
Dietary Fiber 0g	**0%**
Sugars 5g	
Protein 5g	

Vitamin A 4%	•	Vitamin C 2%
Calcium 15%	•	Iron 4%

*Percent Daily Values are based on a 2,000 calorie diet.
Your Daily Values may be higher or lower depending on
your calorie needs:

		Calories: 2,000	2,500
Total Fat	Less than	65g	80g
Sat Fat	Less than	20g	25g
Cholesterol	Less than	300mg	300mg
Sodium	Less than	2,400mg	2,400mg
Total Carbohydrate		300g	375g
Dietary Fiber		25g	30g

Calories per gram:
Fat 9   •   Carbohydrate 4   •   Protein 4

(Source: U.S. Food and Drug Administration, Center for Food Safety and Applied Nutrition)

Something else you may notice is that the % Daily Value is listed to the right of both total fat and saturated fat in this product. No figure is given for the % Daily Value for trans fat, however. Daily Values are dietary reference points for nutrient intakes to help consumers gauge how a serving of a particular food fits into their diets. In the case of saturated fat, the Daily Value is based on a reference diet of 2,000 calories and an uppermost saturated fat intake of 20 grams per day. In the case of vitamins and minerals, the Daily Value refers to target recommended intakes of those nutrients, given a reference diet of 2,000 calories. The % Daily Value indicates the proportion of the day's intake that one serving of the particular product provides.

In this example, one serving of the product contains 5 grams of saturated fat, which amounts to 25 percent of the upper recommended limit of 20 grams per day, assuming a 2,000 calorie diet. Whether that is a lot or a little really depends on what else you may eat in the course of the day and how many servings of this product you eat. It is possible to eat a food high in saturated fat, trans fat, or cholesterol and to balance it out by eating foods very low or devoid of these nutrients throughout the rest of the day.

In general, though, if a serving of a product provides 5 percent or less of the Daily Value for a nutrient, that's low. When it comes to saturated fat or cholesterol, low is good. More than 20 percent is high. When it comes to calcium or vitamin C, higher is better. In this example, then, the product is high in saturated fat, since one serving provides well over 20 percent of the Daily Value for saturated fat.

The trans fat content of the food also matters. The decision to include a Daily Value for saturated fat but not for trans fat is an inconsistency in the labeling regulations, though the FDA had a reason for not stating a Daily Value for trans fat: Because there is no need for trans fat in the diet *and* there is no amount that can be said to be safe to eat, no upper limit could be declared valid. There is no safe upper limit for saturated fat, either, of course, but a Daily Value for it has long been in place on labels.

Working Within the System

The nutrition labeling system isn't perfect, but with the addition of trans fat to the nutrition label, there is enough information to work with. Here's how:

We know the amount of trans fat in the diet is at least as important as the amount of saturated fat in the diet. Therefore, the most practical way to gauge how the trans fat content of a food fits into your diet is to add up both the saturated and trans fat totals and compare that figure to the Daily Value for saturated fat. In other words, count trans fat as you would saturated fat. When you compare similar products, add saturated fat and trans fat, and choose the product with the lowest combined amount.

You should also know the following:

◆ If the total amount of trans fat in a food is less than 0.5 gram per serving and no label claims are made about fat, fatty acids, or cholesterol, the trans fat content of the food does not have to be listed on the nutrition facts label. In that case, the label includes a footnote that states: "Not a significant source of trans fat."

◆ In some cases, partially hydrogenated oil may be listed on a product's ingredient list, but the nutrition facts panel doesn't list any trans fats or the amount is listed as zero. The reason is that it is possible for the amount of trans fat contributed by the partially hydrogenated oil to total less than a half gram per serving. In that event, the food company can round down to zero or opt not to list trans fat at all and to use the required footnote instead. Many brands of peanut butter offer good examples of this.

◆ The labeling regulations apply to dietary supplements as well as food, so if dietary supplements contain more than a half gram of trans fat, the amount must be listed on the supplement facts panel of the product. Some energy bars and nutrition bars, for example, contain trans fats, saturated fats, and/or cholesterol.

Let's Read Some Labels!

Nutrition facts panels on food packages can vary in appearance, but they contain the same basic information. The label below is a horizontal version of the standard vertical label. This example is similar to the label on a loaf of bread.

Find the saturated fat and trans fat content of this product and add the grams of fat in each to get a total combined amount. At the far right of this label, in the fine print, you'll see listed the target limit of 20 grams of saturated fat for a reference diet of 2,000 calories. The limit using a reference diet of 2,500 calories is also listed.

In this example, the combined saturated fat and trans fat content of one serving of this product equals 1 gram (0.5 gram of saturated fat plus 0.5 gram of trans fat). One gram divided by 20 grams equals 5 percent. In other words, the combined amounts of saturated fat and trans fat in one serving of this product equal 5% Daily Value. This product is low in saturated fat and trans fat, and it contains no cholesterol.

Nutrition Facts	Amount / serving	% Daily value*	Amount / serving	% Daily value*	* Percent Daily values are based on a 2,000 calorie diet. Your daily values may be higher or lower depending on your calorie needs:		
	Total Fat 1.5g	**2%**	**Total Carbohydrate** 26g	**9%**		Calories: 2,000	2,500
Serving Size 2 slices (56g)	Saturated Fat 0.5g	**3%**	Dietary Fiber 2g	**8%**	Total Fat	Less than 85g	80g
Servings per container 10	*Trans* Fat 0.5g		Sugars 1g		Sat Fat	Less than 20g	25g
Calories 140	**Cholesterol** 0mg	**0%**	**Protein** 4g		Cholesterol	Less than 300mg	300mg
Calories from Fat 15	**Sodium** 280mg	**12%**			Sodium	Less than 2,400mg	2,400mg
					Total Carbohydrate	300g	375g
					Dietary Fiber	25g	30g
	Vitamin A 0% • Thiamin 15%	Vitamin C 0% • Riboflavin 8%	Calcium 6% • Niacin 10%	Iron 6%			

The label on the next page shows the nutrition facts panel on a package that contains multiple products. In this case, the package contains three individual boxes of breakfast cereal. As you can see, all of these cereals are free of saturated fat, trans fat, and cholesterol.

Nutrition Facts

	Wheat Squares Sweetened		Corn Flakes Not Sweetened		Mixed Grain Flakes Sweetened	
Serving Size 1 Box	(35g)		(19g)		(27g)	
Servings Per Container	1		1		1	
Amount Per Serving						
Calories	120		70		100	
Calories from Fat	0		0		0	
	% Daily Value*		**% Daily Value***		**% Daily Value***	
Total Fat	0g	**0%**	0g	**0%**	0g	**0%**
Saturated Fat	0g	**0%**	0g	**0%**	0g	**0%**
Trans Fat	0g		0g		0g	
Cholesterol	0mg	**0%**	0mg	**0%**	0mg	**0%**
Sodium	0mg	**0%**	200mg	**8%**	120mg	**5%**
Potassium	125mg	**4%**	25mg	**1%**	30mg	**1%**
Total Carbohydrate	29g	**10%**	17g	**8%**	24g	**8%**
Dietary Fiber	3g	**12%**	1g	**4%**	1g	**4%**
Sugars	8g		6g		13g	
Protein	4g		1g		1g	
Vitamin A	0%		10%		10%	
Vitamin C	0%		15%		90%	
Calcium	0%		0%		0%	
Iron	10%		6%		20%	
Thiamin	30%		15%		20%	
Riboflavin	30%		15%		20%	
Niacin	30%		15%		20%	
Vitamin B6	30%		15%		20%	

* Percent Daily values are based on a 2,000 calorie diet. Your daily values may be higher or lower depending on your calorie needs:

	Calories:	2,000	2,500
Total Fat	Less than	65g	80g
Sat Fat	Less than	20g	25g
Cholesterol	Less than	300mg	300mg
Sodium	Less than	2,400mg	2,400mg
Potassium		3,500mg	3,500mg
Total Carbohydrate		300g	375g
Dietary Fiber		25g	30g

In the next example, nutrition information is given for the mix alone as well as for the finished product. There is no cholesterol in the dry mix, but when prepared, the product is a substantial source of cholesterol, probably from the added eggs. Notice that the saturated fat content of this product also increases when prepared according to package directions.

One serving—¼ cup—of the dry mix contains 1 gram of trans fat. Since no % Daily Value is given for trans fat, there is no information provided in this label to indicate how much additional trans fat, if any, the finished product may contain. You might assume that if the recipe calls for milk and eggs, the trans fat content would increase slightly, since there is a small amount of trans fat in animal products. The addition of margarine or solid shortening would likely also increase the trans fat content of the finished product, but liquid vegetable oil, which is trans-fat-free, would not.

Nutrition Facts

**Serving Size 1/12 package
(44g, about 1/4 cup dry mix)
Servings Per Container 12**

Amount Per Serving	Mix	Baked
Calories	190	280
Calories from Fat	45	140

	% Daily Value**	
Total Fat 5g*	**8%**	**24%**
Saturated Fat 2g	**10%**	**13%**
Trans Fat 1g		
Cholesterol 0mg	**0%**	**23%**
Sodium 300mg	**13%**	**13%**
Total Carbohydrate 34g	**11%**	**11%**
Dietary Fiber 0g	**0%**	**0%**
Sugars 18g		
Protein 2g		

Vitamin A	0%	0%
Vitamin C	0%	0%
Calcium	6%	8%
Iron	2%	4%

* Amount in Mix
** Percent Daily values are based on a 2,000 calorie diet. Your Daily Values may be higher or lower depending on your calorie needs:

	Calories:	2,000	2,500
Total Fat	Less than	65g	80g
Sat Fat	Less than	20g	25g
Cholesterol	Less than	300mg	300mg
Sodium	Less than	2,400mg	2400mg
Total Carbohydrate		300g	375g
Dietary Fiber		25g	30g

The next example shows the nutrition facts panel on a small package. Add the saturated fat (1 gram) and trans fat (0.5 gram) and divide by 20 (the number of grams of saturated fat that is the uppermost limit for someone consuming a 2,000 calorie diet). One serving of this product provides about 8% Daily Value when trans fat is added to saturated fat, and the Daily Value for saturated fat is used to assess both. There is less information contained on this label than others, and the figure of 20 grams is one we remembered from previous examples.

Remember, too, that if your calorie intake is less than 2,000 calories per day, you'll need to adjust the levels of intake for saturated and trans fats downward as well. For example, if your calorie intake is 1,500 per day, you'd need to reduce your upper intake limit by 25 percent (since 1,500 calories is 25 percent less than 2,000 calories), giving you an upper limit for saturated fat and trans fat combined of 15 grams per day. Less is even better, assuming you are eating a nutritious diet and getting all the nutrients you need.

Nutrition Facts

Serving Size 1/3 cup (56g)
Servings about 3
Calories 90
  Fat Cal. 20

*Percent Daily Values (DV) are based on a 2,000 calorie diet

Amount/serving	%DV*	Amount/serving	%DV*
Total Fat 2g	3%	**Total Carb.** 0g	0%
Sat. Fat 1g	5%	Fiber 0g	0%
Trans Fat 0.5g		Sugars 0g	
Cholest. 10mg	3%	**Protein** 17g	
Sodium 200mg	8%		
Vitamin A 0% • Vitamin C 0% • Calcium 0% • Iron 6%			

On the next page is another example of a label you may find on a small package. The same basic information is provided, but in a different format.

Nutrition Facts Serv. Size: 1 package, Amount Per Serving:
Calories 45, Fat Cal. 10, **Total Fat** 1g (2% DV), Sat. Fat 0.5g (3% DV), *Trans* Fat 0.5g,
Cholest. 0mg (0% DV), **Sodium** 50mg (2% DV), **Total Carb.** 8g (3% DV), Fiber 1g
(4% DV), Sugars 4g, **Protein** 1g, Vitamin A (8% DV), Vitamin C (8% DV), Calcium
(0% DV), Iron (2% DV), Percent Daily Values (DV) are based on a 2,000 calorie diet.

(Source: U.S. Food and Drug Administration, Center for Food Safety and Applied Nutrition)

Use the information provided on nutrition facts panels to compare the combined saturated fat and trans fat contents of similar products. Choose products with the lowest combined amounts of saturated and trans fats, and also look for foods that are lowest in cholesterol. Evaluate all three of these factors when you comparison shop.

Making Sense of Ingredient Lists

The new regulation requiring trans fat to be listed on the nutrition facts panel largely takes the guesswork out of evaluating packaged foods. Prior to the regulation's taking effect, shoppers had to guess, based on a product's ingredient list, whether or not the food contained trans fat.

Ingredients on food labels are listed in the order of their predominance in the product. As a rule of thumb, ingredients listed first or second usually make up at least half of the product. Herbs and spices are often listed last, because they are used in much smaller amounts.

When solid shortening or partially hydrogenated vegetable oils are listed on a product label, you know that ingredients containing trans fats were used in the food. If these ingredients are near the top of the list, they likely were used in substantial amounts. In that case, the number of grams of saturated fat and trans fat they contribute should show up in the nutrition facts panel on the package. As mentioned earlier, though, food companies sometimes use only very small amounts of ingredients that contain trans fat. The amount may be so small that the number of grams per serving equals less than a half gram. In those cases, you may see partially hydrogenated oil, for example, in the ingredient list but no trans fat listed on the nutrition facts panel.

It also bears repeating that it is important to keep the total picture in mind when assessing the fat content of foods. Trans fat is unhealthy, but so is saturated fat. It is important to keep your cholesterol intake low as well. The goal is to choose foods low in all three and not to replace foods high in trans fat with foods that are high in saturated fat. For example, don't replace margarine, which is high in trans fat, with butter, which is high in saturated fat.

Part II of this book has tips to help you lower your intake of both trans fat and saturated fat as well as cholesterol.

When the Information Isn't There

There may be times when you'd like to know the trans fat content of a food but don't have access to a nutrition facts label. That can happen for a couple of reasons.

Some foods are not required to have a label at all. You won't find nutrition labeling on fresh produce, for example, or on foods in the bakery case. You also won't find nutrition labels on many of the foods you eat at restaurants, food stands, or deli counters. In all these cases it is more difficult to get information about the potential trans fat content of foods as well as saturated fat and cholesterol.

It takes time to acquire the knowledge and skills to know how to choose best in cases like these. Part II of this book focuses on helping you build these skills, and you can use the nutrition counter in Part III to help you estimate the trans fat, saturated fat, and cholesterol contents of foods without labels.

Chapter 4

Putting It All Together

In *Alice's Adventures in Wonderland* by Lewis Carroll, the Cheshire cat and Alice have this exchange:

> "Where are you going?" the cat said.
> "I don't know."
> "Well, either road will get you there."

It is important to have a clear understanding of what your goal is. If you don't know where you want to go, you can't make a plan for getting there. And without some forethought concerning what you need to do to get to your goal, you are less likely to achieve it.

We hear lots of dietary advice these days: Eat more fiber and foods rich in antioxidants. Eat less salt and sugar. Eat enough of some kinds of fats and cut back on others. Buy organic. It can be a challenge to understand which bits of advice to heed, how to prioritize dietary recommendations, and how to put it all together in one neat package of a diet.

This chapter helps explain how advice about trans fat fits within the context of all other dietary recommendations. You learn how you can craft an approach to dealing with diet that is right for you, where you can find some added support, and tips for getting started.

Trans Fat in Perspective

There is no single piece of dietary advice that by itself is enough to ensure the healthiest diet. A collection of recommendations is required that addresses the way we eat now and practical steps we can take to make improvements over time.

The U.S. Department of Agriculture and the U.S. Department of Health and Human Services jointly produce the Dietary Guidelines for Americans, a set of dietary recommendations for the general public that gives advice on how best to eat to support health and reduce the risk of chronic disease. The recommendations are revised every five years based on scientific evidence and the guidance of a committee of nutrition science experts. You can view the Dietary Guidelines for Americans online at www.healthierus.gov/dietaryguidelines/.

Like the regulation requiring trans fat labeling on food packages, the Dietary Guidelines for Americans aren't perfect. Similar to food labeling regulations, the guidelines include input from many stakeholders, some of which stand to lose should Americans significantly alter their eating habits. For this reason, and because nutrition science is complex and is hard to deliver in neat bits of advice, the Dietary Guidelines are not as clear and specific as many people would like. Despite the flaws, they are a helpful point of reference for most people. Here are some key recommendations from the most recent edition of the Dietary Guidelines:

♦ Consume less than 10 percent of calories from saturated fat and less than 300 milligrams per day of cholesterol. Keep trans fat consumption as low as possible.

◆ Keep total fat intake between 20 percent and 35 percent of calories, with most fats coming from sources of polyunsaturated and monounsaturated fats such as fish, nuts, and vegetable oils.

◆ When selecting and preparing meat, poultry, dry beans, and milk or milk products, make choices that are lean, low-fat, or fat-free.

◆ Limit intake of fats and oils high in saturated and/or trans fats, and choose products low in such fats and oils.

These recommendations are in addition to numerous others. To put advice about trans fats into perspective, it is important to understand the bigger picture of the number of ways in which most of us should change our patterns of diet and physical activity. Key recommendations include the following:

◆ Eat a variety of nutrient-dense foods and beverages within and among the basic food groups while choosing foods that limit the intake of saturated and trans fats, cholesterol, added sugars, salt, and alcohol.

◆ Meet recommended intakes within energy needs by adopting a balanced eating pattern such as the USDA Food Guide or the DASH Eating Plan. (DASH stands for Dietary Approaches to Stop Hypertension. More details are available online at www.nhlbi.nih.gov/health/public/heart/hbp/dash/new_dash.pdf.)

◆ To maintain body weight in a healthy range, balance calories from foods and beverages with calories you burn through daily activity.

◆ To prevent gradual weight gain over time, make small decreases in food and beverage calories and increase physical activity.

◆ Engage in regular physical activity and reduce sedentary activities to promote health, psychological well-being, and an appropriate body weight.

- To reduce the risk of chronic disease in adulthood, engage in at least thirty minutes of moderate-intensity physical activity, in addition to your usual activity, at work or home on most days of the week.
- For most people, greater health benefits can be obtained by engaging in physical activity of more vigorous intensity or longer duration.
- To help manage body weight and prevent gradual unhealthy body weight gain in adulthood, engage in approximately one hour or more of moderate- to vigorous-intensity activity on most days of the week but do not exceed caloric intake requirements.

- Achieve physical fitness by including cardiovascular conditioning, stretching exercises for flexibility, and resistance exercises or calisthenics for muscle strength and endurance.
- Eat a sufficient amount of fruits and vegetables while staying within energy needs. Two cups of fruit and 2½ cups of vegetables per day are recommended for a reference 2,000-calorie intake, with higher or lower amounts depending on the calorie level.
- Choose a variety of fruits and vegetables each day. In particular, select from all five vegetable subgroups (dark green, orange, legumes, starchy vegetables, and others) several times a week.
- Consume three or more ounces of whole-grain products per day; the rest should be recommended grains coming from enriched or whole-grain products. In general, at least half the grains should come from whole grains.
- Consume 3 cups per day of fat-free or low-fat milk or equivalent milk products.
- Choose fiber-rich fruits, vegetables, and whole grains often.
- Choose and prepare foods and beverages with little added

sugars or caloric sweeteners, such as amounts suggested by the USDA Food Guide and the DASH Eating Plan.

♦ Reduce the incidence of dental cavities by practicing good oral hygiene and consuming less frequently foods and beverages that contain sugar and starch.

♦ Consume less than 2,300 milligrams of sodium (approximately 1 teaspoon of salt) per day.

♦ Choose and prepare foods with little salt. At the same time, consume potassium-rich foods such as fruits and vegetables.

♦ Drink alcoholic beverages sensibly and in moderation, which is defined as up to one drink per day for women and up to two drinks per day for men.

♦ Some individuals should not drink alcoholic beverages, including those who cannot restrict their alcohol intake, women of childbearing age who may become pregnant, pregnant and lactating women, children and adolescents, individuals taking medications that can interact with alcohol, and those with specific medical conditions.

♦ Alcoholic beverages should be avoided by individuals engaging in activities that require attention, skill, or coordination such as driving or operating machinery.

Still more recommendations address food safety concerns as well as offer advice tailored to the needs of groups with special needs.

How Trans Fat Recommendations Fit In

How do recommendations for trans fat stack up against everything else we're supposed to be doing? In the simplest sense, avoidance of trans fats is compatible with all other dietary advice. In general, dietary guidelines are steering all of us toward a diet that relies less on processed, packaged foods and more on foods as close to their natural state as possible, with special emphasis on foods of plant origin such as fruits, vegetables, beans, peas, nuts, seeds, whole grains, and—for those who consume dairy products and meats—nonfat dairy products and fish. These foods are the foundations of a healthy diet, and they are low in saturated fat, trans fat, and cholesterol.

Working to cut the trans fat out of your diet helps you meet several complementary dietary recommendations—changes that relate to factors that can improve and support good health. For example, we know that heart disease is the leading cause of premature death and disability in our country. Trans fat, saturated fat, and cholesterol in the diet raise the risk for heart disease, while components of fruits, vegetables, legumes, and whole grains protect against it and promote health.

Throughout Part II of this book you will find tips for getting the trans fat out of your diet that are compatible with all other dietary changes you should make to promote health.

Strategic Planning for Your Diet

As individuals we all have different styles of doing things. There is no one right way to go about making dietary changes. The key is to find an approach that works for you and helps you succeed.

With that said, most people find that they fare best when they aim for gradual changes in lifestyle. Where diet is concerned, in particular, it can take time to master new shopping, planning, and cooking skills, to get educated about the science of nutrition, and to establish healthier new traditions to replace some of the old. Taking your time to make dietary changes can be less disruptive to your routine and may help ensure that changes will stick.

So how slow should you go? It's up to you. But like writing a term paper or completing any large project, it can help to break up the task into smaller pieces and focus on one piece at a time.

Part II of this book has eight sections, one on each aspect of the task or area of your diet. That is one way to approach getting the trans fat out. Read each chapter, give yourself some time to master the kinds of changes discussed, and then move on to the next chapter and a new set of challenges. Alternatively, you may decide another approach works better for you. You may want to create a monthly plan, for example, that breaks up the job into assignments such as reading, experimenting with ingredient substitutions in recipes, shopping for trans-fat-free products, meal planning, researching menus at your favorite restaurants, and so on.

You might also find it helpful to take inventory of the foods that are staples in your home. Make a list of the items in your pantry, cupboards, fridge, and freezer. Read food labels and flag items that are high in trans fat, saturated fat, or cholesterol. Then use Part III of this book to identify the remaining foods for which you have no label information but that are likely sources of trans fat.

Once you have identified foods in your home that are high in trans fat, saturated fat, and cholesterol, you can begin to find replacements. Again, Part III of this book can help you find similar products that are more healthful choices. Use the information in Part III to do some comparison shopping without having to leave home. However you decide to move ahead with making dietary changes, think it through and choose an approach that is right for you, your lifestyle, and the people who live with you.

Getting Support, Getting Started

It is important to think about sources of support you can turn to whenever you attempt to make lifestyle changes, including major changes in diet. Sources of support can be friends and family members who are interested in the same issues or just committed to helping you succeed; organizations that offer information or services; community groups that meet to discuss issues and may even offer grocery store tours or cooking classes; and other sources of information such as books, cookbooks, newsletters, and Web sites.

Many good resources are available to help you make changes in your diet and lifestyle. Some—including online diet assessment tools—offer support in the short run by helping you resolve questions or problems quickly, giving you feedback on how you're doing, or providing the incentive to keep going. Others, such as books and other print materials, are good sources of long-term support.

In the accompanying box are a few of my favorite resources to help you get started. Some pertain specifically to the topic of trans fat, but others are more comprehensive and include information about the changes that most of us need to make in our total diet in addition to reducing our intake of trans fat.

Online Dietary Assessment Tools

NutritionQuest
http://nutritionquest.com/freetools/index.htm

This fat screener and fruit and vegetable screener are available free of charge. These simple quizzes take less than five minutes each to complete and provide helpful feedback on saturated fat, fiber, and fruit and vegetable intake for the reduction of cancer and heart disease risks. The researchers who developed these tools also offer a more comprehensive tool which can be ordered via the Web site; its results are similar in accuracy to those obtained through detailed food diaries. The larger quiz takes about thirty minutes to complete using pencil and paper, and it costs $15.

NIBBLE
www.umass.edu/nibble/ratings/queslist.htm

This is a nutrition information site sponsored by the University of Massachusetts–Amherst. A collection of simple quizzes gives feedback on your levels of sugar, sodium, and fat intakes.

CSPI's Rate Your Restaurant Diet
www.cspinet.org/nah/quiz/index.html

This quiz from the Center for Science in the Public Interest is useful for assessing how you do when you are away from home.

Online Weight Management Tools

NHLBI body mass calculator
http://nhlbisupport.com/bmi/

Calculate your body mass index, or BMI—an indicator of total body fat—by using this online calculator from the National Heart, Lung, and Blood Institute.

Cornell calorie calculator
www-users.med.cornell.edu/~spon/picu/calc/beecalc.htm

If you find you need to lose weight, Cornell University maintains this handy calculator for determining the number of calories you need each day to maintain your current weight. To lose a pound a week, subtract 500 calories.

Baylor College's children's BMI percentile-for-age calculator
www.kidsnutrition.org/bodycomp/bmiz2.html

For assessing kids' weights, use this Baylor College of Medicine site for a tool that calculates children's BMIs and provides guidance on interpreting the results.

Baylor College's kids calorie calculator
www.kidsnutrition.org/consumer/nyc/vol1_03/energy_
calculator.htm#

This Baylor site calculates kids' energy needs and offers a list of other resources on handling children's weight problems.

Online Trans Fat Information

U.S. Food and Drug Administration

The U.S. Food and Drug Administration maintains Web sites that offer consumer information on trans fat. See "What Every Consumer Should Know About Trans Fatty Acids" at www.fda.gov/oc/initiatives/transfat/q_a.html as well as "Questions and Answers About Trans Fat Nutrition Labeling" at www.cfsan.fda.gov/~dms/qatrans2.html. More information can also be found at the Web site of FDA's Center for Food Safety and Applied Nutrition at www.cfsan.fda.gov/~dms/transfat.html.   *(continues)*

Harvard School of Public Health's "Nutrition Source"
www.hsph.harvard.edu/nutritionsource/

The Harvard School of Public Health maintains an online health letter, Nutrition Source, that has excellent information on a variety of diet- and health-related topics including fats and cholesterol.

Print Materials

CSPI's "Nutrition Action Healthletter"
www.cspinet.org/cgi-bin/join.cgi

The Center for Science in the Public Interest publishes Nutrition Action Healthletter, one of the most progressive and reliable sources of information on diet and health. Subscription information can be found at the CSPI Web site.

Newspapers

Several major newspapers do a particularly good job with stories that address issues of diet, health, and food policy. Notable ones include stories by Marian Burros and Kim Severson of the *New York Times*, Tara Parker-Pope of the *Wall Street Journal*, and Elizabeth Weise of *USA Today*. My own column, "On the Table," also runs weekly in the *News & Observer* in Raleigh, North Carolina, and in the *Charlotte Observer*, and it appears on my Web site, www.onthetable.net.

Community Resources

Natural foods stores

In addition to being trans-fat-free zones stocked with many good product choices, natural foods stores frequently offer store tours, cooking classes or demos, and lectures by local nutritionists and other health professionals. If there is a natural foods store in your neighborhood, inquire about the availability of these services for the public.

Libraries

Your public library is a good place to find videos, magazines, cookbooks, and other books on topics relating to cuisine, diet, and health. One good choice is *Eat, Drink, and Be Healthy: The Harvard Medical School Guide to Healthy Eating* by Walter C. Willett, M.D. (Free Press, 2005).

Mail Order Sources of Healthy Foods

The Mail Order Catalog
www.healthy-eating.com

The Mail Order Catalog's products include textured vegetable protein and soy foods; substitutes for eggs, cheese, and other dairy products; dried bean flakes; nut butters; organic flours and grains; and others. You'll find free recipes, too.

Pangea
www.pangeaveg.com

Pangea's products include trans-fat-free cookies and baked goods, meat and dairy substitutes, and baking supplies. The site sells gift baskets, too.

Getting the Trans Fat Out

Getting the junk out of your kitchen—and moving good stuff in—is vital to setting up a trans-fat-free environment. In this part of the book we'll cover ways to get the trans fat out of your refrigerator and pantry by focusing on all the grocery categories where trans fats typically hide. We'll not only cover what you *shouldn't* eat but also include tips and suggestions for products that are *good* choices and will help squeeze the trans-fatty foods out. Note that while we'll cover a lot of ground, some food categories aren't specifically addressed. Beverages, for example, don't typically harbor trans fat, so they're generally not addressed here, although soft drinks and full-fat dairy drinks are certainly not healthful choices.

We'll also discuss meal planning and preparation ideas to help make trans-fat-free living easier to achieve. Once your home is in order, we'll turn our focus to the choices you have when you eat out. The ultimate goal is to help eating remain pleasurable while avoiding harmful trans fat and maintaining a diet that supports health.

Let's get started!

Chapter 5

Get the Trans Fat
Out of Your Kitchen

Healthy lifestyles begin in the kitchen. That's because, for most of us, the majority of our meals come out of our homes, whether we eat there or carry a lunch or snack to school or the office.

There is a huge potential advantage to eating food you make at home rather than meals purchased outside: control. Buying healthy ready-made foods and ingredients can help ensure that what you put on the table or in the lunch box will support health and not undermine it.

Furthermore, the more you make *from scratch* at home, without relying on commercially prepared foods, the easier it is to eat well and avoid harmful trans fat. Ready-made processed foods and restaurant menus are often loaded with trans fat, saturated fat, sodium, and added sugar. When you cook with fresh whole ingredients at home, meals are likely to be lower in these ingredients.

And when you cook at home and eliminate these harmful elements, everyone benefits. Studies show that kids who eat meals prepared at home normally eat more fruits and vegetables than kids who eat a diet of mainly prepackaged or commercially prepared meals. They eat less trans fat, saturated fat, and fried foods, and drink fewer soft drinks. Their diets are higher in calcium, fiber, folic acid, iron, and vitamins B and E.

You know that cooking for yourself and your family is a good thing to do, but you might be thinking, "Who has time?" There is a key to pulling off home cooking these days when most of us are so busy. The essential factor is simplicity. It's a concept I've grown to appreciate. One champion of simplicity in the kitchen was Helen Nearing, a woman I met in 1995, shortly before she was killed in a car accident at the age of ninety-one. She was a legend in some circles, having been a pioneering homesteader with her husband, Scott, in New England and having lived there since the 1930s.

Helen gave me a copy of one of her books, *Simple Food for the Good Life: An Alternative Cook Book* (first published in 1980 and reissued by Chelsea Green Publishing Company in 1999). A phrase on the front cover of the book makes me laugh and captures the attitude I so admired in Helen: "Intended for the use of people of moderate fortune who do not affect magnificence in their style of living." Elsewhere in the book she states that her objectives are to "write on simple food for simple-living people" and to pass on her ideas about cooking "which call for little experience, little time, little money, few ingredients and a minimum of complication."

Helen subscribed to the no-recipe approach to cooking. "I rarely read or consult a cookbook," she said. "I'm a spur-of-the-moment cook and make do with what materials are at hand."

She was on to something. Keeping the right things "on hand" is, of course, another key to successfully preparing healthy trans-fat-free meals at home.

In this chapter we'll take an in-depth look at what it takes to create a kitchen that contains the supplies that best allow you to prepare meals that are free of unhealthy ingredients. We'll cover ways to be more efficient, equipment to have on hand to make meal preparation easier, staples to stock, and where to buy them.

Tricks of the Trade

1. **Start by cleaning up.** A clean, well-organized, well-stocked kitchen will give you peace of mind and make it much easier and more pleasurable to cook. You'll know what you have and what you don't, and everything will be easier to access. Deep-clean. Remove everything from cupboards, drawers, and pantry, and get rid of anything you don't use: appliances, old party supplies, paper goods that have been collecting dust, and any items that don't belong in the kitchen but have made their way into your cupboards anyway. Throw them away, put them in a garage sale pile, or donate them to charity. You'll free up space so that items you do use are accessible. Empty the cabinets and drawers a few at a time and wash them inside with soap and hot water. Pull out but don't replace cupboard and drawer liners. Crumbs and bugs like to hide under their edges. Throw away any foods in your refrigerator and freezer that have been sitting unused for a long time or that are out of date. Purge your cupboards and pantry of any foods you know you won't use. They're taking up space and are a distraction.

2. **Get organized.** Over time, you may have shelved items out of place or piled baking sheets, pots, pans, and lids in unwieldy piles in your cabinets. Take them out, rearrange them, and store them in such a way that they are easy to see and reach. If you need more space, consider buying an overhead rack for pots and pans that can hang from your ceiling or kitchen wall. You might also consider adding a baker's rack or a movable island on wheels with extra drawers and shelves for storage. Label jars and canisters of baking supplies. Unless you use huge quantities, buy oils and spices in small containers so that you can replace them more often and know they're fresh. That way they also take up less cupboard space.

3. Remember to clean as you go. Who wants to face a pile of dirty dishes after dinner? Make that mountain a molehill by putting away supplies; rinsing utensils and equipment, and placing them in the dishwasher; and wiping down the sink and countertops while you cook.

4. Use select convenience foods. You'll pay more if someone peels your carrots for you, but the extra cost can be worth it if you know that having already-peeled carrots will make it easier for you to cook and therefore to eat healthy food. Good choices are minced garlic in a jar, prechopped veggies for stir-fry, and prewashed salad greens. More about convenience foods will be found in upcoming chapters. It bears repeating: Eating more meals prepared at home from plain whole foods is an important strategy in weeding the trans fat out of your diet. Prepared fruits and vegetables can be big time-savers.

5. Make more than you need. Double the recipe and freeze chili, lasagna, muffins, and cookies made with trans-fat-free ingredients. You'll have meals and snacks ready to reheat on days when you haven't the time or inclination to cook.

6. Recycle. Stir leftover cooked greens into lentil soup and serve cooked beans or vegetable ratatouille over leftover steamed rice or couscous. Always keep your healthy leftovers; you'll be surprised at how many uses you can find for them in other dishes.

7. Combine creatively. Toss dried cherries and sunflower seeds into a mixed green salad. Add chopped walnuts, diced pears, and cinnamon to cooked oatmeal. Make burritos with black beans and mashed sweet potatoes. Add a handful of corn to a pot of chili.

8. **Try one-dish meals** if you're in a hurry or don't have much energy for cooking. They're convenient and quick to fix, and are much healthier than frozen entrees and packaged foods, which are more likely to contain saturated and trans fats. A large salad, hearty soup, casserole, or pasta dish can be all you need. Use lots of color, which is easily done if you add several vegetables. A chunk of good whole-grain bread on the side may round out the meal.

9. **Become a Sunday cook.** Monday or Tuesday is also fine. Just pick a time to fix two or three foods that can be eaten over the next few days or frozen for later. Spend the time on cooking when you have it or when you're in the mood, and save time and hassle later when it may be less convenient.

10. **Take stock of your kitchen habits.** Notice what your habits are in the kitchen and look for shortcuts. Identify ways to make life a little easier and meal preparation more enjoyable. You'll cook more of your meals at home that way and be less likely to lean on commercial products that contain trans fat and saturated fat.

Tools of the Trade

11. **Supply yourself with the utensils and appliances you need to work efficiently,** but don't get bogged down with too many gadgets that you don't use. If your countertop is jammed with small appliances, you won't have enough counter space to work on. For example, I prefer to use an old-fashioned crank can opener that I store in a drawer, so I have one less appliance on my counter. And not everybody needs a big countertop mixer;

some people can make do with a handheld mixer, and some don't use a mixer at all, only a whisk. Think about your lifestyle and equipment needs, and then pare down wherever possible so that you don't waste money and kitchen space. That said, here is some basic equipment to consider having on hand:

- Spatulas, wooden spoons, whisks
- Measuring cups and spoons
- Mixing bowls in various sizes
- A good set of kitchen knives, including a paring knife, a serrated knife, a French chef's knife for chopping vegetables, and a bread knife
- Countertop or handheld mixer
- Slow cooker (such as a Crock-Pot)
- Heavy-duty blender or juicer
- Baking pans and sheets
- Food processor
- Pots and pans in assorted sizes

12. Consider whether a rice cooker would be helpful. I love it. It allows you to steam rice while doing something else rather than watching the stovetop to ensure the rice doesn't boil over. Prices range from $30 to $300 depending on capacity and quality. Rice is a good foundation for many healthy home-cooked dishes, so I find this particular appliance very useful.

13. You might also consider a pressure cooker. When you're under time constraints and need to fix fast, healthy meals, a pressure cooker can produce in ten minutes what would otherwise take two hours. Pressure cookers can slash cooking time by two-thirds or more. They allow you to have lentil soup ready in seven minutes, risotto in five. You can cook casseroles, stews, curries, and chili in the time it takes to set the table. Those frightening, rickety, jiggle-top contraptions your mother may have had are a thing of the past. Newer models, including brands such as Mirro and Presto, are designed with features that prevent excessive pressure from building up and are safer to use. And now even better second-generation pressure cookers, introduced in Europe and available in the United States, have numerous advantages over first-generation types. Their features include stationary pressure regulators to replace the old removable jiggle-tops. Brands include Kuhn Rikon, Magefesa, and Zepter. All are available online or in specialty stores, and prices range from $20 to $300 or more.

14. Keep a few extras of some items on hand. While not essential, they can make your meals look special and enhance the enjoyment of eating at home so you might eat at home more often. Something as simple as some new cloth napkins, coordinating placemats, or a tablecloth can brighten a table. Consider a few beautiful serving dishes such as a pottery bowl or two-tiered plate. I have a decorative iron trivet that stands on legs about eight inches high. I use it to serve pizza that I assemble at home using crust made from whole wheat flour brushed with olive oil. Decorative spreaders and serving spoons or forks can also be fun.

15. Keep a few good cookbooks on hand. You may not want anything fancy, but you should have recipes for simply prepared wholesome foods. You might consider *Great Vegetarian Cooking Under Pressure* by Lorna Sass (William Morrow, 1994), Didi Emmons's *Vegetarian Planet* (Harvard Common Press, 1997), and my own *Vegetarian Cooking for Dummies* (Wiley, 2001). Why vegetarian? Vegetarian cookbooks tend to make greater use than conventional cookbooks of a wider range of trans-fat-free plant ingredients, such as beans, whole grains, and vegetables. You'll also find that more olive oil is used and less butter. You'll still need to watch out for recipes that rely heavily on eggs and fatty dairy ingredients such as cheese, but without meat-based entrees, the saturated fat and cholesterol loads of vegetarian meals tend to be much lower.

Tasteful Techniques

16. Use vegetable oils and trans-fat-free soft margarines (the kind that come in liquid or spray forms, or in a tub) for all your cooking needs. The combined amount of trans fat and saturated fat they contain is less than the amount in solid shortening, stick margarine, butter, and other forms of animal fat. you can match the type of oils with the recipe. Olive oil, for instance, has a strong delicious flavor best suited to savory rather than sweet dishes. Similarly, the distinctive flavor of walnut oil mixed with vinegar goes well on salad greens.

17. Colorize your plate. It's a simple way to boost the nutrient and flavor punch of your diet. Fruits and vegetables deeply pigmented in bright colors (or white) are packed with needed nutrients and are free of those you don't need, such as trans fat. In contrast, many foods high in trans fat are dull in color (think of cookies and doughnuts). Colorful foods tend to have high concentrations of healthy vitamins and other substances, including beneficial phytochemicals, that help protect against coronary artery disease and some forms of cancer. Visualize a dinner plate with a bright and flavorful mix of dark leafy greens topped with red tomatoes, sliced onions, grated carrots, and diced green peppers alongside a black bean and sweet potato–filled burrito topped with salsa and a sprig of parsley. It sounds colorful and delicious, and it's very healthy as well. This "keep it colorful" approach really works: If you eat at least eight servings of nutrient-dense fruits and vegetables each day, you'll be sure to get enough dietary fiber, vitamins, minerals, and phytochemicals. At the same time, those healthy foods will likely displace the junky and trans-fat-filled food you might otherwise have eaten.

18. Use herbs and spices liberally. Fresh or dried, plain herbs and spices such as nutmeg, cardamom, cinnamon, basil, oregano, mint, rosemary, cumin, and a hundred others add richness and flavor to foods and can keep you interested in healthy recipes.

19. Use infused oils. These are vegetable oils that have been steeped in herbs or fruit essences, so they carry that flavor into whatever dish they're used to make. For instance, blood orange–infused olive oil is delicious on salads, and vegetable oil infused with rosemary tastes great when brushed on oven-roasted potatoes.

Supermarket Savvy

20. Rotate your shopping trips among several stores. If you go to the same store each week, you may become bored or begin to dread the task of grocery shopping. Instead, vary it. In addition to your neighborhood supermarket or natural foods store, occasionally include ethnic food markets, farmers' markets, and specialty shops on your itinerary in order to keep your shopping routine interesting and to introduce fresh ideas and interesting products to your kitchen.

21. Give yourself extra time on your first trip to a natural foods store. Repeat the produce section ritual and roam every aisle, looking carefully at what's on the shelves in each aisle. Then pick up a few products to sample. As always when you try new things, you'll find some you won't like, but you'll stumble upon some new favorites, too. Here are a few of my favorite things to buy at natural foods stores, where you can find them all free of trans fat and saturated fat.

22. *Fortified soy milk.* It's often sold in aseptic shelf-stable boxes. Anyone who is lactose-intolerant or who wants to avoid the fat found in most dairy products should try soy milk. (Or, if you're allergic to soy, try fortified rice milk instead.) It can be used, cup for cup, in all the same ways as cow's milk. Experiment with brands to find the one you like best. If you grew up drinking cow's milk, it might take a little while to grow accustomed to the subtly different taste of soy milk or rice milk. But after a few weeks most people grow to love it, and switching can cut a major source of saturated fat from your diet. I buy vanilla-flavored soy milk for cereal or to drink straight, but the plain flavor is versatile because you can also use it in mashed potatoes and cream soups.

23. *Breakfast cereals.* The brands at natural foods stores are all made with whole grains, and some are sweetened with fruit juice. They have no partially hydrogenated oils, so they're trans-fat-free. There are some great choices for kids, too. Well-known brands include Barbara's Bakery, Arrowhead Mills, Grainfield, Kashi Company, Health Valley, Hain, and Lifestream.

24. *Tempeh.* This is a food made from whole cultured soybeans; it is sold in half-inch slabs in the refrigerated or frozen foods section of the store. It's a traditional Indonesian food. I cut it into one-inch cubes and sauté it with greens in a soy-ginger sauce.

25. *Powdered vegetarian egg replacements.* This product works wonderfully in virtually any recipe that calls for eggs, and a one-pound box lasts a long time. It's a mixture of vegetable starches that is not only trans-fat-free but also free of cholesterol and saturated fat. You'll find it with the baking supplies. My favorite is called Egg Replacer, made by Ener-G Foods.

26. *Instant soups, the cup-of-soup variety,* and other instant products. Just add hot water, and you have soup or chili or noodles or even hot cereal in its own bowl. These products are great for bag lunches. They were actually the forerunners of the brand-name knockoffs. They're made with organically grown ingredients and are much healthier than the sodium-heavy brands you'll find in conventional supermarkets. Fantastic Foods, Just a Pinch, and Nile Spice are a few examples.

27. *Whole-grain mixes.* Natural foods stores carry a wide variety of pancake and quick bread mixes, rice, and cous-cous. These whole-grain dishes and side dishes are similar to their conventional counterparts, but they are lower in sodium and contain no partially hydrogenated oils or unnecessary additives.

28. Prices of natural foods at natural foods stores are often substantially less than prices of the same brands sold in conventional supermarkets. A good example is soy milk, including brands such as Eden Soy, Silk, and Westbrae Natural West Soy. Many supermarkets now carry soy milk, but volume sales in natural foods stores often allow prices to be lower. A practical strategy is to buy certain staples at natural foods stores and supplement them with carefully chosen foods from supermarkets or wholesale club stores.

29. Wholesale club stores such as Costco, Sam's Club, and B.J.'s can be a source of wholesome trans-fat-free foods at substantial cost savings over similar products at conventional supermarkets or natural foods stores. Excellent values for healthy foods at these stores include fresh salsa; fresh pesto; hummus; peanut butter and other nut butters; dried fruits; seeds and nuts; olive oil; vegetable oil sprays; soy milk; veggie burger patties; and whole-grain breads and breakfast cereals. All these are convenient, versatile products for a healthy trans-fat-free lifestyle.

30. Shop with a list and don't shop when you're hungry. That classic Weight Watcher's tip is a good way to avoid impulsive shopping that may result in foods high in bad fats making their way into your shopping cart. (A case can be made for shopping when you're hungry—if you use it as a way to break out of old ruts and increase your receptivity to new, healthy foods. If you try this, take care to read labels for bad fats before you choose.)

31. Be a frequent label reader, particularly at conventional supermarkets. Companies often change the ingredients in products. You won't know this unless you check the labels from time to time.

32. Think through your approach to grocery shopping. Your shopping habits influence what you buy, and what you buy ultimately dictates what you eat. To eliminate trans fat from your diet and eat more healthily in general, you'll need to have the right supplies at home.

33. Maintain a grocery list on your kitchen counter or refrigerator door, and take the list with you when you go to the store. Not only will shopping from a list keep you from forgetting what you went shopping for, but it will also help you maintain control. A list can minimize the chance of going off your plan and impulsively buying foods and ingredients that you don't want to have in the house.

34. If you have difficulty resisting snack foods and treats, which are often loaded with trans fat, be sure to go to the store *after* you've eaten, not before. Going when you're hungry lowers your resistance to temptation and increases the likelihood that you'll make impulsive purchases.

35. Buy monounsaturated and polyunsaturated oils instead of saturated fats, such as butter, lard, and bacon grease, and trans fats, such as solid shortenings and stick margarine. Mono-unsaturated oils include olive, peanut, and canola oils. Polyun-saturated oils include soybean oil, corn oil, and safflower and sunflower oils.

36. For now, it's a good idea to **avoid tropical oils** such as co-conut oil, cocoa butter, and palm kernel oil. Science is still un-certain about the effects that these plant sources of saturated fat have on blood cholesterol levels.

37. Make no assumptions about any food. Read the label. Food companies will be reformulating products for some time to remove the trans fat, and until we have a trans-fat-free soci-ety (not likely anytime soon!), you'll have to be vigilant about checking the label on every single thing you buy. Remember, even if the trans fat has been removed from one product in a brand line, you can't assume that it has been removed from other products of the same brand.

38. Also remember that **foods labeled as trans-fat-free can still be poor choices** if they are high in saturated fat. In some cases, manufacturers who remove trans fat from their products may choose to replace it with other solid shortenings high in saturated fat. Treat saturated fat exactly as you do trans fat: Get it out!

39. Stay alert to the products most likely to contain trans fat: commercial baked goods such as pies, cookies, muffins, cakes, pastries, and crackers, as well as margarine.

40. Shop for foods in a variety of forms. Fresh is often best, but it's not always convenient. Plan to stock a range of fresh, frozen, canned, and packaged foods.

41. The very best fruits and vegetables are locally grown, in season, and fresh. Frozen produce runs a close second. Canned can be practical, and despite some nutrient losses due to heating and time on the shelf, they can still make a sizable contribution to your nutritional bottom line. Buy reduced-sodium canned veggies when they are available. Use the color trick to ensure variety: red tomatoes, pink peaches, yellow corn, green broccoli, purple chard, white cauliflower.

42. Spend extra time in the produce section of the store. Walk up and down the aisles and take the time to notice all the different types of produce available. Most people bypass the majority of the items in the produce area—the healthiest products in the store. They make a beeline for what they know well, such as iceberg lettuce, bananas, and maybe some tomatoes. Does this sound like you? If so, take a risk and buy an item or two that you've never tried before. You may discover a new favorite food.

43. Use color as a guide to getting the widest range of nutrient-dense foods. Colored gelatin and multicolored marshmallows in breakfast cereal don't count, of course. Fresh fruits and vegetables in their just-picked form are always free of trans fat and saturated fat. For example:

> **44.** *Red:* tomatoes, watermelon, strawberries, red bell peppers, beets, red grapes, radishes, red onions

> **45.** *Orange and yellow:* apricots, peaches, cantaloupe, oranges, sweet potatoes and yams, mangoes, papayas, acorn and butternut squash

> **46.** *Green:* broccoli, green bell peppers, green beans, kiwifruit, green grapes, peas, avocados, leafy greens such as spinach, kale, Swiss chard

> **47.** *White:* bananas, daikon radishes, onions, cauliflower, garlic, white potatoes, leeks, turnips

48. *Blue and purple:* blueberries and blackberries, plums, raisins, purple and black grapes, eggplant, purple endive

49. Legumes—dried beans and peas as well as lentils—**are highly nutritious and versatile.** Combine several—garbanzos, pintos, red kidney beans, and white kidney beans—to make many-bean chili. Mash them for dips, soups, and spreads. Combine them with rice, pasta, and other grains to make interesting entrees. You can buy them dried in bags or in bulk, and you can sort, soak, and cook them. For convenience, you can also buy them canned. Before using canned beans, rinse them in a colander to remove most of the added salt.

50. Seeds and nuts are packed with protein, healthy oils, and beneficial phytochemicals. Sprinkle walnut halves or sunflower seeds on salad, add slivered almonds to steamed vegetables, or toss a handful of cashews into a pot of chili. Commercial brands of peanut butter usually list partially hydrogenated oil on the ingredients list, but check out the nutrition information. The amount of trans fat in peanut butter is usually negligible.

51. Breads, cereals, and other whole grains can be a great accompaniment to a meal—try a slice of whole-grain bread or a couscous salad—or they can be the backbone of an entree such as rice pilaf or a plate of spaghetti. Leftover rice and other cooked grains can be reheated and served with steamed vegetables or topped with chili; as a filling for bean burritos, tacos, or cabbage rolls; or used to make rice pudding.

52. When you shop for whole unprocessed grains and products made primarily from whole grains, look for natural product brands. The natural foods stores have the best selection by far, but many conventional supermarkets also carry store-brand natural and organic products that are trans-fat-free. Look for these:

- Whole-grain cold and hot breakfast cereals
- Whole wheat pasta in different shapes
- Several varieties of rice, such as jasmine, Arborio, bas-mati, and brown
- Whole-grain breads, rolls, flour tortillas, waffles, and muffins
- Unusual grains, including ancient ones such as ama-ranth, spelt, quinoa, kamut, teff, buckwheat, oats, and millet

Shopping Alternatives

53. **Increasing the amount of fresh produce in your diet** is a smart way to squeeze *out* many of the commercially prepared products that contribute unwanted trans fat and saturated fat. There are several alternatives to supermarkets for good-quality fresh fruits and vegetables during the growing season.

54. Receive your fruits and vegetables the same day they're picked by **joining a CSA (community supported agriculture) farm.** Here's how it works: Residents of a community pay a local farmer a predetermined amount of money before the growing season. In return, they get a portion of the harvest throughout the season. There are only about one thousand CSA farms in the United States, but the number is growing. The specifics of each CSA arrangement vary. Some farms grow herbs and flowers in addition to vegetables and a limited amount of fruit. Subscribers usually receive an agreed-upon weekly portion; usually it's enough for a family of four, or about six pounds. Some farms offer half portions. Subscribers usually collect their food at a central pickup point. Costs vary, too, but expect to pay several hundred dollars for about thirty weeks of produce, which is similar to what you would pay for the same or even lower quality produce at the supermarket. Some CSA farms give a discount if you pay early or send them a new subscriber. Online information and lists of CSA farms in your state can by found by searching the Web or through state cooperative extension offices or farm stewardship associations.

55. **Shop for locally grown seasonal produce** at roadside stands and farmers' markets. Small farmers need your support, and the fruits and vegetables they grow are incredibly good for your health. Locally grown seasonal fruits and vegetables are more nutritious because they come to your table within a day or even hours of being picked. That preserves vitamins that otherwise would deteriorate in the days it takes foods to be shipped across country and stocked in supermarkets. Plus, fresh, in-season foods taste better. Produce trucked cross-country is often picked before it has fully ripened.

56. **Consider installing a kitchen garden at your home.** You need a sunny spot to grow tomatoes and peppers, but a big backyard isn't mandatory. If you don't have a lot of space, try container gardening: You can use a few clay pots, an old barrel, or a planter. Good choices for many backyards include bell peppers, lettuce, radishes, carrots, green onions, green beans, and cherry tomatoes or the full-size variety. (Most garden shops now carry tomato plant varieties cultivated to grow in containers on patios.) For larger gardens where plants can spread out, try cucumbers, zucchini, pumpkins, cantaloupe, and watermelon. You can also tuck some plants, especially herbs, here and there between shrubs and flowers in the yard; try parsley, chives, basil, and rosemary.

Chapter 6

Get the Trans Fat Out of Bread and Breakfast

As we all know, Mom was right about a lot of things. One of them was the importance of eating breakfast. Research has shown that children who eat breakfast perform better in school. That's no surprise. It's hard to focus on the three Rs when another R—rumbling stomach—is interfering. There is no doubt that we all perform better when we have enough energy. As anyone with diabetes or hypoglycemia will tell you, regular meals can make the difference between feeling well and feeling poorly.

But there is still another good reason to eat breakfast: Breaking the fast as you begin a new day may help control your appetite and the quality of your diet throughout the day. In fact, a 2003 Harvard University study found an association between breakfast and lower rates of obesity. Adults who ate breakfast were found to be up to 50 percent less likely to be obese compared to people who skipped breakfast.

Think about it. How do you feel when you get to work or school on an empty stomach? Does hunger lead you to a vending machine? Eating at home—even if it is nothing more than a bowl of cereal or a slice of toast and juice—can ward off intense late-morning hunger and make it less likely that you'll eat something you'd be better off without.

Of course, as previously mentioned, eating healthy at home isn't always easy. One challenge is finding the time to eat in the morning. And what if you're not hungry before it's time to head out the door? Yet another challenge is keeping healthy and quick foods on hand.

The time snag can be dealt with in several ways. Do what makes sense for you. That may mean setting the alarm fifteen minutes earlier to give you time to eat a bowl of cereal or a piece of fruit. Some people find it helpful to set out a bowl and a box of cereal the night before. Or grab toast and fruit to eat at your desk or on the go.

What if you just can't tolerate a meal first thing in the morning? My suggestion is to have a two-part breakfast. Drink a glass of fruit juice or eat a piece of fresh fruit before you leave the house. Then take the second part of your breakfast with you to eat a little later in the morning. Good portables are fresh fruit, a whole-grain muffin, a slice of bread with peanut butter, or a cup of nonfat yogurt.

That leaves the challenge of knowing which breakfast foods are trans-fat-free and good for you. Many breakfast foods are notoriously full of trans fat. Topping the list of trans-fat-heavy morning terrors are biscuits, croissants, doughnuts, pastries, and eggs and hash browns grilled in shortening (the customary practice at most restaurants).

That's what this chapter is all about: showing you which foods to pile on your plate for morning meals that will satisfy you and provide you with that morning boost most of us need to perform our best throughout the day. We'll cover strategies for avoiding breakfast trans fat and finding suitable substitutes. What can you have for breakfast if the foods you have traditionally turned to are off the menu? Plenty. Read on.

Breads and Spreads

57. When you choose a spread for your toast, bagel, or other breakfast bread, compare product labels carefully. Add the number of grams of both saturated fat and trans fat, and choose the product with the lowest total of combined bad fat. In the example that follows, the best choice is the tub margarine, which has a combined saturated fat and trans fat total of 1.5 grams. Always go for the lowest total possible since there is no safe level of intake of either saturated fat or trans fat.

Compare Spreads!
Keep an eye on saturated fat, trans fat, and cholesterol!*

Nutrition Facts	Nutrition Facts	Nutrition Facts
Serving Size 1 Tbsp (14g)	Serving Size 1 Tbsp (14g)	Serving Size 1 Tbsp (14g)
Servings Per Container 32	Servings Per Container 32	Servings Per Container 32
Amount Per Serving	Amount Per Serving	Amount Per Serving
Calories 100 Calories from Fat 100	Calories 100 Calories from Fat 100	Calories 60 Calories from Fat 60
% Daily value	% Daily value	% Daily value
Total Fat 11g 17%	Total Fat 11g 17%	Total Fat 7g 11%
Saturated Fat 7g ◄━ 35%	Saturated Fat 2g ◄━ 10%	Saturated Fat 1g ◄━ 5%
Trans Fat 0g ◄━	Trans Fat 3g ◄━	Trans Fat 0.5g ◄━
Cholesterol 30mg ━► 10%	Cholesterol 0mg ━► 0%	Cholesterol 0mg ━► 0%

Butter†	**Margarine, stick‡**	**Margarine, tub‡**
Saturated Fat: 7g	Saturated Fat: 2g	Saturated Fat: 1 g
+ Trans Fat: 0g	+ Trans Fat: 3g	+ Trans Fat: 0.5g
Combined Amt.: 7g	Combined Amt.: 5g	Combined Amt.: 1.5g
Cholesterol: 10% DV	Cholesterol: 0% DV	Cholesterol: 0% DV

*Nutrient values rounded based on FDA's nutrition labeling regulations. Calorie and cholesterol content estimated.

†Butter values from FDA Table of *Trans* Values, January 30, 1995.

‡Values derived from 2002 USDA National Nutrient Database for Standard Reference, Release 15.

(Source: U.S. Food and Drug Administration, Center for Food Safety and Applied Nutrition; accessed on December 26, 2005, at: www.cfsan.fda.gov/~dms/transfat.html)

58. Examples of tub margarines that are trans-fat-free and low in saturated fat include Organic Smart Balance Whipped Buttery Spread (2.5 grams of saturated fat per tablespoon) and Canoleo Soft Margarine (2 grams of saturated fat per 14 grams, or about one tablespoon).

59. In lieu of margarine or butter on toast and other breakfast breads, use a little jam, jelly, or honey. They're trans-fat-free.

60. Another good toast topper is baked beans. It's a British tradition, and a healthy one at that. Beans are rich in protein and fiber, and they're trans-fat-free.

61. More good toast toppers are apple butter, nonfat cottage cheese mixed with cinnamon and sugar, a dollop of cherry or blueberry conserves, and nonfat cottage cheese mixed with apple butter, cherries, or blueberries. You don't need all the sugar; each of these choices is delicious and can be a great Danish pastry stand-in!

62. Biscuits, croissants, doughnuts, pastries, and deep-fried fast-food breakfast items such as French toast strips and fried pies are chock-full of trans fats. Good substitutes include bagels, whole-grain breads, English muffins, and homemade muffins and quick breads made with vegetable oil. It is still a good practice, though, to read labels on any products sold in conventional supermarkets and compare brands, since breads vary in trans fat content.

63. If you buy breads from in-store bakeries, ask store personnel for ingredient and nutrition information if it isn't provided on the bread bag. Like restaurant foods, bakery items are not required to carry nutrition and ingredient information.

64. Fruited bagels are naturally slightly sweet and make a good substitute for doughnuts and breakfast pastries. Try apple cinnamon, cinnamon raisin, blueberry, and cranberry bagels.

65. Looking for a good spread for bagels that is free of trans fat and very low in saturated fat? Try this one, which is made with tofu. It has a consistency and texture similar to whipped cream cheese. Use this not-overly-sweet topper on toast, English muffins, and French toast. This recipe is from my book *Vegetarian Cooking for Dummies* (Wiley, 2001).

Maple Nut Spread

PREP TIME: 15 MINUTES

COOKING TIME: 40 MINUTES

Yield: 2 cups, or about 8 servings

⅓ *cup raisins or currants*

½ *cup hot water*

½ *cup firm tofu*

¼ *cup low-fat yogurt*

½ *cup pure maple syrup*

½ *teaspoon cinnamon*

1 *tablespoon sesame tahini*

2 *tablespoons pure vanilla extract*

2 *teaspoons all-purpose flour*

⅓ *cup chopped walnuts*

1. Preheat the oven to 350 degrees. Use vegetable oil to lightly grease a 1-quart baking or casserole dish.

2. Place the raisins or currants in a small bowl or cup and pour the hot water over them. Set aside to soak.

3. Place the tofu, yogurt, maple syrup, cinnamon, tahini, vanilla, and flour in a food processor or blender. Blend well, stopping frequently to scrape down the sides. Turn the ingredients with a spatula if necessary to facilitate thorough blending.

4. Drain the raisins and chop them into small pieces or give them a whirl in a food processor. Add the raisins and walnuts to the tofu mixture and stir well.

5. Pour the tofu mixture into the baking dish and bake, uncovered, for 40 minutes, or until set. Cool completely before serving.

66. **To make an aromatic and nutritious topping for French bread rounds or homemade rolls,** smear a whole roasted clove of garlic on them. Here's how: Preheat the oven to 350 degrees. Pull the loose outer layers off a bulb of garlic, leaving enough so that the cloves remain intact. Use a sharp knife to cut off the top quarter inch, exposing the tops of the cloves inside, and drizzle them with a couple of teaspoons of olive oil. Wrap the bulb loosely in aluminum foil, seal the foil completely, and place in the hot oven. Bake for 1 hour, or until the cloves are soft. Remove from the oven and place the bulb in a serving dish. Smear the softened garlic on bread. If the cloves are hard to spread, squeeze the bulb to loosen them.

67. Muffins sold in most supermarkets contain large amounts of trans fat. The good news is that muffins are quick and easy to make at home and store in the freezer until you need them.

68. One of my all-time favorite homemade muffin recipes is one I adapted from the Moosewood Collective's *Moosewood Restaurant Book of Desserts* (Clarkson Potter, 1997). These muffins are trans-fat-free and very low in saturated fat. They'll disappear in about a day.

Easy Banana Muffins

PREP TIME: 10 MINUTES
COOKING TIME: 20 MINUTES

Yield: 12 muffins

½ cup vegetable oil
1 cup packed brown sugar
1 tablespoon Ener-G Egg Replacer (found at natural foods stores) or 4 egg whites beaten lightly and 4 tablespoons water
3 cups mashed bananas (about 3 large bananas)
2 cups all-purpose flour or 1 cup white and 1 cup whole wheat
1 teaspoon baking powder
1 teaspoon baking soda
¼ teaspoon salt
2 teaspoons pure vanilla extract
½ cup chocolate chips and/or ¼ cup chopped nuts (optional)

1. Preheat the oven to 350 degrees and oil a 12-cup muffin tin or use a paper liner.
2. In a large bowl, hand mix the oil, sugar, egg replacer and water, and mashed bananas until smooth.
3. Add the flour, baking powder, baking soda, salt, and vanilla, and stir until blended.
4. Stir in the chocolate chips and/or nuts if desired.
5. Spoon the batter into the muffin cups and bake for about 20 minutes, or until the tops are browned. Cool before serving.

Egg Alternatives

69. Steer clear of all forms of fried eggs served in restaurants, since nearly all restaurants grease egg pans and griddles with trans-fatty butter or solid shortening. At home you can use olive oil or another vegetable oil instead.

70. Controlling your intake of saturated fat and cholesterol goes hand in hand with cutting out trans fat, so **look for ways to eat fewer eggs** or eat only egg whites and avoid the yolk, the storehouse for cholesterol. Egg whites are cholesterol-free. You can use egg whites in place of whole eggs in omelets. Just remember that in recipes, two whites are equal to one whole egg. You can also use egg substitutes such as EggBeaters and buy small or medium eggs instead of large eggs.

71. Substitute tofu for eggs in "tofu scrambler," a dish similar to scrambled eggs but low in saturated fat and free of trans fat and cholesterol. You can use hot or cold scrambled tofu as a sandwich filling in a pita pocket or on a hoagie roll. This simple recipe is from *Being Vegetarian for Dummies* (IDG Books Worldwide, 2001).

Peppers and Tofu Scrambler

PREP TIME: 10 MINUTES

COOKING TIME: 10 MINUTES

Yield: 4 servings

2 tablespoons olive oil
1 medium onion, chopped
2 teaspoons minced garlic
2 cups bell pepper strips (green, red, yellow, or mixed)
Two 12-ounce bricks of firm tofu
½ teaspoon black pepper
1 teaspoon turmeric
1 tablespoon soy sauce
Salt to taste

1. Heat the olive oil in a large skillet over medium heat. Add the onion, garlic, and bell peppers and cook, stirring occasionally, until the onions are translucent and the peppers are soft, about 8 minutes.

2. Crumble the tofu into the bell pepper mixture. Add the black pepper, turmeric, soy sauce, and salt, and mix together with a wooden spoon or spatula. Heat thoroughly, mixing and scrambling the ingredients continuously, for about 2 minutes.

Breakfast Specialties

72. Hold the butter and margarine and instead **top waffles and pancakes with warm maple syrup or fruit conserves.** They're trans-fat-free and low in total fat.

73. **Make waffles and pancakes at home when you have the hankering.** I know I'm repeating myself, but it's important to remember that restaurants use large quantities of trans-fat-filled shortening and artery-clogging butter to grease griddles, waffle irons, and egg pans. Eat these foods at home instead where you can control the methods used to make them.

74. **My favorite pancake recipe** is an old family favorite my mother made when we were kids. She called them Healthy Pancakes. On Saturday mornings we'd ask her to make us some "healthies." Cook these pancakes as soon as possible after mixing the batter to ensure light and fluffy pancakes. These pancakes contain zero trans fat, very little cholesterol, and only 1 gram of saturated fat per pancake. Leftovers keep well in the refrigerator for a few days and can be reheated in a microwave oven.

Healthy Pancakes

PREP TIME: 10 MINUTES
COOKING TIME: 5 MINUTES

Yield: 6 servings or about twelve 5-inch pancakes
1 cup whole wheat flour
½ cup white flour
⅓ cup wheat germ
1 teaspoon baking soda
1 tablespoon baking powder
1 teaspoon cinnamon
½ teaspoon salt
1¾ cups skim milk, vanilla soy milk, or rice milk
¼ cup vegetable oil
1 egg or EnerG Egg Replacer or 2 egg whites
2 egg whites, beaten stiffly

1. Place the flours, wheat germ, baking soda, baking powder, cinnamon, and salt the in a medium-sized bowl.

2. Add the milk, oil, and egg and stir well, using a whisk. Break up any remaining chunks of flour by using the back of a spoon.

3. Fold in the beaten egg whites with a wooden spoon or rubber spatula. The batter will be thick but light and somewhat foamy.

4. Pour a ⅓-cup measure of batter onto a hot oiled skillet (canola or corn oil work well). When the pancakes are bubbly all over and the edges are browned, turn them over and cook on the remaining sides for about 30 seconds, or until the undersides are browned. Serve immediately.

75. **Another griddle classic is French toast.** At fast-food restaurants, French toast sticks are deep-fried and therefore laden with trans fats. At other restaurants, French toast is made on greasy griddles with trans-fat-heavy butter, which is as bad for you as fried. The recipe below is a variation on French toast that is popular with strict vegetarians, or vegans, because it contains no eggs, milk, or butter. It is not your mother's French toast, but it is free of trans fat, saturated fat, and cholesterol. Most important, it is delicious and nutritious.

Easy 'n' Healthy French Toast

PREP TIME: 10 MINUTES
COOKING TIME: 5 MINUTES

Yield: 4 servings

2 large, ripe bananas
1 cup plain or vanilla soy milk or rice milk or regular skim milk
¼ teaspoon ground nutmeg
½ teaspoon pure vanilla extract
8 slices whole-grain bread
Powdered sugar
Pure maple syrup, warmed
Sliced bananas or strawberries for garnish

1. In a blender or food processor, puree the bananas, milk, nutmeg, and vanilla. Pour the mixture into a shallow pan such as a pie tin, cake pan, or an 8 by 8-inch baking dish.
2. Generously oil a griddle and heat it until a drop of water spatters when flicked onto the surface.

(continued)

3. Dip both sides of each slice of bread into the milk mixture and transfer each slice to the griddle. The first side will take about 2 minutes to brown. Turn gently and carefully, because the bread has a tendency to stick to the griddle. Cook the second side for about 3 minutes.

4. Carefully remove the French toast from the griddle and turn it so that the brown side is faceup. Dust each slice with powdered sugar and serve with warm maple syrup. Garnish with fruit slices and serve.

Breakfast Cereals

76. **Read carefully the nutrition facts label on boxes of breakfast cereal.** The trans fat content of different brands—and different varieties of the same brand—can vary. Manufacturers also may change the ingredients. You may not notice unless you check the label periodically.

77. **Go for the whole grain.** Dietary recommendations issued by the federal government recommend that we eat at least three servings (about 3 ounces) of whole grains each day. That means at least half of the cereals and breads we eat every day should be made from whole grains. How do you know a whole grain when you see one? The easiest way is to read the food label and look for one word: whole—whole wheat, whole rye, whole oats, and so on. Ingredients are listed in order of their predominance in the product. If whole wheat is the first ingredient listed, it probably makes up at least half of that product. Don't be tricked by imposters. "Wheat flour" is *refined* white flour. If it were whole, it would say so. And just because the bread is brown doesn't mean it's made from whole wheat. It could be caramel coloring. Check the label.

78. A good way to meet dietary recommendations for whole grains is to **start each day with a big bowl of cold or hot whole-**

grain cereal—at least one cup. Cereal makes a good snack, too. Here are some good trans-fat-free choices, but there are many others in Part III of this book.

BONUS TIP: COLD CEREALS

Barbara's Brown Rice Crisps
Familia Muesli
General Mills Cheerios or Wheat Chex
General Mills Fiber One
Healthy Choice Toasted Brown Sugar Squares
Kashi-brand Kashi
Kellogg's All-Bran
Kellogg's or Post Raisin Bran
Post 100% Bran or Bran Flakes
Post Shredded Wheat
Quaker Puffed Wheat
U.S. Mills Uncle Sam
Weetabix

BONUS TIP: HOT CEREALS

Arrowhead Mills 4-Grain Plus Flax
Arrowhead Mills 7 Grain
Arrowhead Mills Cracked Wheat
Arrowhead Mills Oat Bran
Kashi Breakfast Pilaf
Quaker Old-Fashioned or Instant Oats
Roman Meal Cream of Rye
Roman Meal Multi-Grain
Wheatena

79. Keep a variety of whole-grain dry cereals on hand. You can mix two or three for a little variety.

80. Set up a slow cooker at night and fix breakfast while you sleep. Old-fashioned or quick-cooking oats can be varied by adding slivered almonds, chopped walnuts and dates, dried fruit, diced Granny Smith apples, fresh blueberries, nutmeg, cinnamon, vanilla, maple syrup, or brown sugar.

81. **Your morning bowl of oatmeal** benefits greatly if you fold in leftover baked apples. Also good in oatmeal are stewed apples, applesauce, or stewed prunes.

82. **Expand the number of hot cereals you eat beyond ol' reliable oatmeal.** Other good choices include Roman Meal Instant Cream of Rye, Mother's Oat Bran, and multigrain blends sold in natural foods stores and supermarkets.

83. **If you can't eat cereal at home, take breakfast to work.** Individually packaged hot cereal cups (add hot water, stir, let sit for a few minutes, and enjoy) are trans-fat-free. Brands include Fantastic Foods and Dr. McDougall's Instant Hot Cereals.

84. **Mix granola** (make sure it's trans-fat- and saturated-fat-free), **Post Grape-Nuts, or other dry cereals with nonfat or soy yogurt or cinnamon applesauce,** or serve cereal and yogurt or applesauce in layers, parfait style, in a glass cup.

Bonus Tip: Add a tablespoon of wheat germ to cold or hot cereals. It's rich in vitamin E, zinc, and B vitamins.

Nontraditional Breakfasts

85. **Try miso soup,** which is a traditional breakfast food in Japan. It is a delicious broth-based soup made by adding hot water, diced tofu, and scallions to miso, which is a thick, fermented paste made from soybeans. It is high in sodium but trans-fat-, saturated-fat-, and cholesterol-free.

86. **Smoothies can serve as a nutritious breakfast** when you have to grab and go on busy mornings. Make your own in a blender or food processor using whatever ingredients you have on hand—vanilla soy milk, fruit juice, fresh fruit, frozen berries, nonfat frozen yogurt, or a few tablespoons of maple syrup—as a sweetener. To make an Orange Julius you'll need 1 cup orange juice, 2 cups frozen nonfat vanilla yogurt, 1 teaspoon pure vanilla extract, and five or six ice cubes. Place all ingredients in a blender and process on high speed for about one minute. Add more or less orange juice to achieve the consistency you prefer. Pour into a cup and be on your way. For another alternative, blend 1 cup vanilla soy milk, half of a ripe banana, 1 cup frozen mixed berries, and 2 tablespoons pure maple syrup.

87. Save those leftovers and eat them for breakfast the next morning. Leftover bean burritos, pesto pasta, bean chili, and other nutritious entrees can make an encore appearance the next morning. See Chapter 8 for more details.

88. An all-fruit breakfast can be a good way to start the day. Fruit is easy to digest and provides quick energy. Scoop the seeds from a cantaloupe half and fill the half with berries or sliced bananas and a dollop of nonfat vanilla yogurt as a garnish. Fruit salad tossed with fresh mint leaves, made the day before and chilled overnight, is another refreshing option.

89. Watch out for breakfast bars, toaster pastries, and energy bars. Many have bad fat lurking inside. Read labels carefully to screen out those with trans fat or a high combined total of trans fat and saturated fat.

Breakfast Beverages

90. Freshly squeezed fruit juices are a vitamin-packed treat. One of my favorite juice blends is an equal mixture of freshly squeezed orange juice and fresh carrot juice. I squeeze my own oranges at home or use a not-from-concentrate carton juice, but I usually buy the fresh carrot juice in my supermarket or local natural foods store. You can adjust the proportions of orange and carrot juices to suit your preference. Either way, it's a nutritional powerhouse of a drink.

91. Instant cocoa mixes bought at the supermarket may contain hydrogenated vegetable oils. **Make your own trans-fat-free hot cocoa simply at home.** This one is easy to make:

Creamy Homemade Hot Cocoa

PREP TIME: 1 MINUTE
COOKING TIME: ABOUT 8 MINUTES

Yield: 6 servings

⅓ cup unsweetened cocoa powder (available in any supermarket)
⅓ cup sugar
1½ cups water
4½ cups plain or vanilla soy milk or rice milk
½ teaspoon pure vanilla extract

1. Combine the cocoa powder, sugar, and water in a 3-quart saucepan. Heat until boiling, stirring frequently, and then boil for 2 minutes, stirring constantly.
2. Add the milk and continue stirring until steaming hot.
3. Remove from the heat and add the vanilla. Stir briskly with a whisk before serving.

92. Coffee is a trans-fat-free breakfast staple for many of us. To date, research has found few strong links between coffee and any adverse health effects. Some recent studies have even suggested benefits. If you drink coffee and use a whitener, use skim or 1 percent or 2 percent milk or soy milk instead of saturated-fat-filled whole milk, cream, or nondairy creamers made with partially hydrogenated oils.

93. Silk-brand soy milk is a particularly good whitener for coffee and even hot tea because it's free of trans fat, saturated fat, and cholesterol, and it doesn't curdle when mixed with hot beverages as some other brands of soy milk have a tendency to do. Silk also makes a nondairy creamer specifically for coffee that is fine to use. Both products are sold in supermarkets and natural foods stores.

94. Tea, the most popular beverage in the world, is also trans-fat-free and fine for most people to drink. Like many plants, tea leaves contain flavonoids, which are antioxidants that may reduce damage that occurs naturally to the body's cells over time. Tea, especially green tea, is rich in a group of simple flavonoids called catechins; some research has linked them to lower rates of heart disease and some forms of cancer.

95. Be careful not to drink too much tea. Large amounts of tea can inhibit the body's absorption of iron from meals. Counteract this effect by drinking tea between, rather than with, meals. Vitamin C also helps the body absorb iron, so include good sources of vitamin C—tomatoes, citrus fruits, cabbage, and potatoes—with meals as well. Up to three cups of tea per day is a reasonable intake for tea lovers.

96. Many people in Central America enjoy fresh watermelon juice as a refreshing and nutritious drink any time of day. Toss chunks of cold ripe watermelon into a blender and give them a whirl. Add a little water or fruit juice (pineapple, orange, or lime) if necessary to create the consistency you prefer. For variation, use cantaloupe or honeydew melon.

Chapter 7

Get the Trans Fat Out of Salads, Dressings, and Dips

It's time to turn a new leaf.

Eating frequent and big green salads is a good way to minimize your intake of trans fat, since salads are made with fresh ingredients, lettuce and veggies, that haven't been processed with added fats. The more salad you eat, the more trans-fat-laden foods you're *not* eating. An added bonus is that eating big salads can often help you cut calories and control your weight. A large salad as the main course for one meal a day can cut several hundred calories from your daily diet—enough to help some people shed up to a half pound a week.

All of this assumes, though, that the salad dressings you're using don't add back the fat and calories you dodged by skipping the lasagna or meat loaf. Two tablespoons of some salad dressings, the standard portion listed on product labels, can add up to 200 calories to a meal. Ladle on more, and the mixed greens may as well be a plate of nachos.

But calories aren't the only criterion for a healthy dressing. The best salad dressings are also low in sodium, saturated fat, and trans fat. Only a couple of tablespoons of salad dressing can pack up to 500 milligrams of sodium, more than a third of the amount any of us should have in an entire day. Cheese, eggs, and mayonnaise add saturated fat to creamy dressings such as Roquefort and blue cheese. Most salad dressings are low in trans fat, though you might find some made with partially hydrogenated oils. The main risk with salad dressings is that they contribute saturated fat that increases the combined bad fat in your diet.

Fortunately, it's not necessary to limit yourself to a squirt of lemon juice on your baby spinach leaves. In fact, salad dressings don't have to be a problem at all. There are enough good choices that you should be able to stay interested in eating salad most days of the year. In this chapter we'll cover strategies for adding more trans-fat-busting salads to meals, along with health-supporting trans-fat-free dressings that are also low in saturated fat. In addition, we'll talk about ideas for dips that can be used to accompany fresh vegetable sticks, crackers, and snack chips.

Salad Days

97. To many people a salad is boring. It means a bowl of anemic iceberg lettuce crowned with a few shreds of carrot, a cucumber slice, and maybe a tomato wedge. **Break away from the iceberg lettuce rut,** and you will find that you're more able to stay interested in salads. Crisp, dark green romaine is a more nutritious choice. Even more flavorful is arugula, a dark, leafy green known for its distinctive sharp, spicy, peppery flavor, similar to that of mustard greens.

98. A good way to ensure that fresh salad materials don't go bad in your refrigerator before you can eat them is to **set aside time right after you shop to preprepare them.** Choose a time when you are relaxed and can spend half an hour or so washing, peeling, and chopping. Put on some good music or park a friend or family member nearby and gab. Just do it. Store prepared lettuce and cut-up veggies in plastic bags and airtight containers in the refrigerator so you have them on hand, ready to use in a salad, for when you are in a hurry or don't want to fuss.

99. Keep cold salads on hand in hot weather. You won't heat up your house by cooking or using the oven. Many salads can be served as a one-plate low-cal meal, too. An added bonus: You won't have to wash as many dishes!

100. Slice fresh strawberries in half and toss them with broken walnuts, baby spinach leaves, and poppyseed dressing. Slices of papaya, mango, and avocado are also good with salad greens.

101. Set aside time on a regular basis to fix fresh salads. Use whatever you have on hand. Here are some good combinations.

> **102.** *Cucumber and tomato salad with diced red onion* (best if eaten within two days).

> **103.** *Greek salad* (also best eaten within two days) made with mixed greens, chopped green pepper, red onion, tomatoes, and cucumbers. Top it with black olives and a sprinkling of crumbled feta cheese.

> **104.** *Melon salad,* and add fresh mint from the garden.

> **105.** *Green bean and boiled potato salad* can use some steamed fresh beans. Toss with vinegar and olive oil. You can add chopped pimentos or roasted peppers.

> **106.** *Vinaigrette coleslaw* with onions, grated carrots, and red cabbage. Try a variation using fresh dill from the garden.

107. One of my all-time favorite salads is a combination of summer garden vegetables. The possibilities are endless: romaine lettuce, green onions, red cabbage, carrots, radishes, tomatoes, bell peppers, and cucumber. Mince them finely and toss well with garbanzo beans, croutons, and creamy Italian dressing for an incredible salad that keeps well in the refrigerator for several days. With a couple of pieces of Italian bread, it's a meal in itself.

108. Make a three-bean salad in the wintertime when your vegetable garden is in hibernation. Here's a quick and easy recipe: Rinse and drain one 15½-ounce can each of cut green beans, cut wax beans, and dark red kidney beans. Place the beans in a large bowl and add ½ cup chopped green bell pepper; ½ red onion, chopped; ½ cup sugar or less, to taste; ⅔ cup vinegar; ⅓ cup vegetable oil; and 2 teaspoons black pepper. Toss and chill overnight. Toss the salad once more before serving.

109. Some good trans-fat-free and saturated-fat-free additions to tossed green salads can add texture, color, and flavor. Great additions include sunflower seeds, pumpkin seeds, walnut pieces, slivered almonds, avocado slices, raisins, dried cherries or cranberries, fresh diced or dried apples or pears, figs, garbanzo beans, dark red kidney beans, grated carrots, pickled beets, shredded red cabbage, and sliced green onions.

110. Try a chopped salad. I've craved these ever since ordering an Italian chopped salad at a restaurant a couple of years ago. It was similar to Middle Eastern fatoush, a version of chopped salad with little bits of pita bread mixed in. The key—and what's so good about it—is that every ingredient in the salad is finely chopped. Use a food processor if you like, though I chop by hand with a French knife. The bonus is that there are no big chunks of broccoli or unwieldy lettuce leaves to flick salad dressing onto your blouse or shirt! Use mixed greens or romaine or whatever you have on hand, plus carrots, bell peppers, celery, black olives, green onions, radishes—whatever you like. I toss mine with raspberry walnut vinaigrette dressing.

Bonus Tip: Sometimes I also like to layer one salad on top of another. Start with a basic mixed green salad, add a big scoop of three-bean salad or vinaigrette coleslaw, and top it all off with a few pickled beets and sunflower seeds.

111. A food processor reduces the work of making salads. Here's a recipe for Confetti Coleslaw, an old family favorite, that takes only minutes to make if you have the help of your trusty appliance. Shred 3 cups cabbage, ½ cup carrots, and ½ cup green bell pepper. In a small pitcher, combine ⅓ cup rice vinegar and 2 tablespoons vegetable oil. Whisk the vinegar and oil together and pour it over the cabbage mixture. Toss, chill, and serve.

Dressed for Success

112. For the all-around healthiest salad dressings, look for the lowest calorie options. Compare brands to find those lower in calories; anything up to about 100 per serving is reasonably healthy. Experiment to find the varieties you like best. Oil-based dressings spread more easily than thick creamy dressings, so you may need less dressing and save calories.

113. Taking dressing "on the side" can also help your salad be healthier. Dip forkfuls of salad into the dressing, and you'll likely use less than if you poured dressing directly on the salad.

114. Buy dressings with the least sodium. Compare brands and make sure that you're using those lowest in sodium. You're doing well if you can hold the sodium to under 200 milligrams per serving.

115. Or try this tangy lemony dressing. Whisk together the juice of half a lemon, 1 tablespoon red wine vinegar, 2 tablespoons olive oil, 2 teaspoons salsa, ¼ teaspoon paprika, and ⅛ teaspoon dried tarragon leaves. Chill and whisk again before serving. Makes two servings, about 120 calories each.

116. I loved the salads my grandmother used to make with lettuce from her garden tossed with plain cider vinegar and oil. **You can't go wrong if you stick with vinegar and oil.** You can vary it today, though, by buying flavored vinegars such as raspberry and tarragon and other varieties including balsamic, red wine, and cider. Try oils flavored with fruit essences or infused with herbs and spices. Walnut oil is another good choice. It has a distinctive flavor that goes well with a salad of fresh baby greens, sliced red onion, tomato, and black olives.

117. Look for dressings with low saturated fat and trans fat. Most salad dressings are relatively low in saturated fat and low or free of trans fat, since vegetable oil is one of the main ingredients. Check labels to be sure and choose those with less than 2 milligrams of saturated fat per 2-tablespoon serving. Some varieties of blue cheese and other mayonnaise- and cheese-based dressings have far more.

118. The Center for Science in the Public Interest has published **a list of the healthiest commercial salad dressings** in its Nutrition Action Healthletter (a great resource that I recommend to all readers). Among the best are Brianna's Lemon Tarragon, Drew's All Natural Raspberry, Ken's Steak House Lite Salsa Ranch and Lite Ranch, Marie's Raspberry Vinaigrette and Red Wine Vinaigrette, and, my personal favorite, Newman's Own Light Raspberry & Walnut.

119. Some of the best salad dressings are the simplest. Even plain blenderized fresh fruit can be light and refreshing over a plate of greens. Acidic fruits work well because they add a zip that can often take the place of salt; for example, peel a tangerine and remove the seeds, break it into sections, and place them in a blender or food processor. Add 1 tablespoon lemon juice and blend until smooth. Serve over fresh mixed baby greens. This one is completely fat-free.

120. **Another easy homemade dressing,** one of my favorites, contains no trans fat and minimal saturated fat. Combine in a small pitcher 1 teaspoon lemon juice (I use the juice of one or two fresh lemon wedges), 1 tablespoon red wine vinegar, 2 tablespoons extra-virgin olive oil, 2 teaspoons salsa, ¼ teaspoon paprika, a sprinkling of freshly minced tarragon leaves (or ⅛ teaspoon dried tarragon leaves), and salt to taste. Mix well and then whisk the ingredients together again before serving over your favorite salad.

121. **Mayonnaise can add saturated fat and cholesterol to salads** such as Waldorf and egg salad. A healthier choice is a mayo-like product made from tofu that is free of trans fat and cholesterol and is low in saturated fat. Examples include Nasoya-brand Nayonaise, Follow Your Heart–brand Vegenaise, and Hain-brand Eggless Mayonnaise. I use tofu "mayo" to make a delicious egg salad substitute (see no. 352, Chapter 10).

122. **Seasoned rice vinegar is a mild yet highly flavorful product that can stand alone as a dressing for many salads.** Find it in the supermarket with other varieties of vinegar or in the Asian food section.

Take a Dip

123. **For a break from salads, serve fresh vegetable sticks**—green peppers, carrots, cucumbers, radishes, broccoli, cauliflower—with bean dip, low-fat salad dressings, or salsa.

124. Hummus is a mouthwatering traditional Middle Eastern bean dip that is also low in bad fats. It's made from garbanzo beans (also known as chickpeas), and if you have never tried it, put it on your "must do" list. Hummus is delicious served cold as a vegetable dip or sandwich filling (and try adding some well-rinsed alfalfa sprouts and grated carrots). Traditionally, it's served warm in a shallow dish with a squeeze of fresh lemon juice and a drizzle of olive oil on top. Wedges of pita bread are used to scoop the dip.

125. You can save money by making your own hummus at home. It's easy. Combine in a blender two 15-ounce cans of garbanzo beans, 2 teaspoons minced garlic, 4 tablespoons sesame tahini (find it in natural foods stores), the juice of one freshly squeezed lemon, and ¼ teaspoon white pepper. Puree and add a few teaspoons of water or extra lemon juice if the mixture is too thick to blend. Serve in a shallow bowl or on a plate. Garnish with small, thin wedges of lemon, black olives, and/or tiny strips of sweet pickle arranged around the edge of the dish. Swirl a few tablespoons of olive oil on top and sprinkle the whole dish with paprika for color. Serve with pita bread wedges that have been brushed with olive oil and lightly toasted in the oven. The recipe makes about four ½-cup servings. The best part is that this recipe contains no trans fat, no saturated fat, and no cholesterol.

126. For a delicious and healthy dip for tortilla chips, mash the meat from one avocado and mix it with ¼ cup diced sweet onion, 1 teaspoon minced garlic, 2 tablespoons fresh lime juice, and 2 tablespoons salsa. Make this dip just before you're ready to serve it, because all the fresh ingredients can make it go bad after only a couple of hours.

127. Nonfat vanilla yogurt makes a good dip for fresh berries and pineapple and melon chunks.

128. Make a spicy dip for crackers and vegetables by whisking together in a small bowl 1 cup plain nonfat yogurt, ¼ cup minced onion, ¼ teaspoon salt, 1 teaspoon chili powder, ½ teaspoon garlic powder, and ½ teaspoon cumin. Chill thoroughly before serving. Leftovers are good on a baked potato.

129. Black bean dip is good with raw vegetable sticks. Then the leftover dip, which thickens as it sets, can be used as a filling for burritos or tacos the next day.

130. Make your own black bean dip! Heat the contents of a 15-ounce can of black beans. Add ½ cup warm water and then mash the hot beans well with a potato masher or fork. Add half of a chopped small yellow onion, 2 teaspoons minced garlic, and ¼ cup salsa. Reheat until the dip is hot and bubbly. Add more water by the tablespoon if needed to achieve the desired consistency.

131. Set out a dipping dish for crusty breads and rolls. At dinnertime, pour a puddle of olive oil onto a plate. Add several tablespoons of balsamic vinegar, a dash of freshly ground black pepper, and a sprinkling of Parmesan cheese. Tear off bite-sized pieces of bread and dip each bite into the olive oil mixture. Divine.

132. Make a sour cream substitute that can be used to top a baked potato or as the base for a dip. Place ½ cup nonfat cottage cheese in a food processor or blender and add 1 tablespoon lemon juice. Process until smooth.

133. You can make the sour cream substitute even healthier by substituting 8 ounces silken firm tofu for the cottage cheese.

Chapter 8

Get the Trans Fat Out of Soups and Sauces

It is possible for soups—and sauces, too—to contain trans fat, but they're more likely to contain substantial amounts of saturated fat. Since we are concerned about the *combined* load of trans fat plus saturated fat in your meals, it pays to spend some time examining soup and sauce dos and don'ts.

But there's a flip side—a positive one—to soups and some sauces. Like big, fresh salads, soups are helpful aids for getting the trans fat out of your diet, because eating more of them will displace foods that otherwise tend to load our plates with unhealthy trans fat and saturated fat. Soup also has one-dish-meal simplicity that makes meal planning and cleanup easy. Make a batch in advance or warm up the ready-made variety. Pair it with some good bread, and it's a meal.

Soup is nutritious, too. Depending on the variety, it can be rich in protein, fiber, vitamins, and minerals. Thick or chunky soups made with beans, potatoes, and other starchy vegetables pack the most nutrients. They are also higher in calories, so they "stick with you" longer than soups with more broth. Examples of thicker soups that are good for you include navy bean, split pea, lentil, chili, corn chowder, squash, and apple, and soups made with pasta and beans.

Soups with a higher proportion of broth tend to be filling but less nutrient-dense and lower in calories. A bowl of broth-based soup in lieu of an entree a few nights each week can be a good strategy if you are trying to lose a few pounds. A few examples are minestrone, Chinese hot and sour or wonton soup, vegetable barley, and alphabet. In general, though, both broth-based soups and heartier soups tend to be relatively low in calories, trans fat, and saturated fat compared to most other entrees.

One of the few drawbacks to soup is that it's typically high in sodium. Excessive sodium intakes can increase your risk of coronary artery disease and stroke. Processed foods and fast food are prime sources. Low-sodium, ready-made soups are available in stores, or you can cut back on salt if you make soup from scratch. Otherwise, balance high-sodium soup by limiting salty foods at other meals and eating fresh fruits, vegetables, and other unprocessed foods more often.

Taking Stock

134. **Don't assume that packaged and ready-to-eat soups are trans-fat-free.** Always read the label. Partially hydrogenated oils are used extensively in processed foods, and they do turn up in commercial soups.

135. **Soup stock, which is the basis for almost any type of homemade soup, is easy to make from scratch.** No recipe is required, and you can use what you have on hand. One way to start is to save the water used to boil a pot of potatoes, greens, cabbage, or any other vegetable. Transfer the liquid to a larger pot, add several more cups of water, and toss in any vegetable scraps or odds and ends you may have: celery leaves, chopped onion, old carrots, and so on. Bring the water to a boil and let simmer for at least two hours. Strain and add salt to taste. Let the broth cool. It can be stored in the refrigerator for three to four days or frozen for several weeks before use.

> Bonus Tip: Freezing broth in ice cube trays is easy and very convenient. Remove the frozen cubes and store them in plastic freezer bags until needed.

136. Broth can also be made by dissolving vegetable bouillon cubes in hot water. Miso paste (see Chapter 6) can also be used as an all-purpose base for broth.

137. If you don't have the time or the inclination to make broth from scratch, **you can get healthy store-bought broth if you know where to look.** Pacific Natural Foods brand makes convenient fat-free vegetable and mushroom broths packaged in shelf-stable, aseptic, one-liter containers. You can buy them at supermarkets and natural foods stores. Always remember to look at the label before purchasing store-bought broth.

138. Avoid soups made with artery-clogging heavy cream or whole milk. If you make cream soup at home, use nonfat milk or plain soy milk instead.

139. Another trick is to puree cooked beans or lentils in a food processor and stir them into a pot of soup for a saturated-fat-free thickener.

140. You can also puree a cooked potato or soft tofu with vegetable broth.

141. There is an almost unlimited variety of healthy soups from which to choose that are not of the cream-based variety, and if you give some attention to how you serve it, the soup meal can continue to be appealing indefinitely.

142. Pair your soup with the right bread. With colorful minestrone, serve a crusty baguette or slice of rustic olive herb bread.

Pair creamy-colored potato and leek soup with marble rye bread or a poppy seed roll.

143. Vary the serving bowl. In addition to cereal bowls, I like to serve soup in pottery mugs and large chili bowls with handles or shallow, rimmed soup bowls.

144. Branch out with ethnic soups. You can find them in natural foods stores and specialty markets, or peruse the Web or library for recipes and make them yourself at home.

145. *African peanut soup.* A friend of mine in West Africa makes hers with sweet potatoes, Granny Smith apples, peanut butter, vegetable broth, olive oil, onion, cumin, cinnamon, and black pepper.

146. *Spanish black bean soup.* Top it with a tablespoon of minced onion.

147. *Chinese hot and sour soup.* This one will clear your sinuses in allergy season or if you have a cold. It's also delicious.

148. *Tortilla soup.* Try it with fresh cilantro and lime juice.

149. Soup is easy to make. You can make it in a slow cooker overnight or while you're away at work, or simmer it on the stove while you do other things. Experiment with ingredients. You can start with any vegetable or bean soup recipe (such as the one listed in tip number 151) and toss in odds and ends from the pantry or refrigerator—a handful of elbow macaroni, small amounts of leftover cooked vegetables, or unused pasta sauce. Stir leftover spinach into lentil soup, for example, or a handful of rice or pasta into a pot of vegetable soup.

150. Soup is one leftover that need not go to waste. Pack whatever you don't finish at dinner and take it to school or work.

151. Soups made with split peas, lentils, or beans don't need a base, since the beans make them so flavorful and thick. Leftover bean soups and chili thicken in the refrigerator. Reheated, they make a good topping for a baked potato. Here's an easy recipe for split pea soup:

Split Pea Soup

PREP TIME: 15 MINUTES
COOKING TIME: 40 MINUTES

Yield: 4 servings

1 cup dried green split peas
4½ cups water
1 large onion
2 medium potatoes
2 celery stalks
½ teaspoon dried marjoram
Salt and freshly ground black pepper to taste

1. Rinse and drain the split peas, then place them in a large saucepan and add the water.
2. Peel and chop the onion and potatoes. Chop the celery, including the leaves. Add them to the split peas and water.
3. Bring the ingredients to a boil over medium heat and simmer until the peas are soft, about 40 minutes.
4. Add the marjoram, salt, and pepper.
5. Remove 2 cups of soup from the pan, puree it in a blender or food processor, and then stir it back into the remaining soup. Serve hot.

152. Soup is the perfect project for a Sunday cook. Make a big batch during the weekend and enjoy it the following week when you do not have the time or energy to cook.

Bonus Tip: One drawback to soup is the high sodium content, especially in commercial brands. If you make your own soup at home, you can leave out added salt entirely. If you do that, or if you buy low-sodium prepared products from the store, consider these tips I received some years back from Robert Pritikin, son of the late diet guru Nathan Pritikin, when I interviewed him for a book about supermarket shopping: "I always add a little Thai hot sauce—particularly if I'm eating a low-sodium soup—or a squeeze of fresh lemon," he said. "It brings out the flavor without adding sodium."

The Scoop on Sauces

153. Be diligent about reading food labels on any sauce you buy at the store. Trans fat can turn up in surprising places.

154. In general, sauces made with dairy products tend to be high in saturated fat, boosting the combined bad fat quotient in your diet. Always avoid cream sauces, Alfredo pasta sauce, Hollandaise, and other rich cream- or cheese-based sauces.

155. Healthy trans-fat-free sauces tend to have fruits and vegetables as their bases. Pourable fruit, for example (mashed blueberry, cherry, and/or apricot), is delicious on pancakes and waffles. Onions, garlic, and other garden staples combine to make versatile sauces and marinades.

156. Use sauces and marinades to perk up cooked vegetables and other foods or to give them character. Cook in them or use them as dips or condiments. Many sauces and marinades are free of trans fat and saturated fat. You can find the following and others like them in gourmet stores, neighborhood supermarkets, natural foods stores, and ethnic markets.

157. Pace Sweet Roasted Onion and Garlic Cooking Sauce

158. Stonewall Kitchen Garlic Rosemary Citrus Sauce

159. Fischer & Wieser Charred Pineapple Bourbon Sauce

160. D. L. Jardine's Killer Barbecue Sauce

161. Consorzio All Natural Jamaican Jerk 10-Minute Marinade

162. Consorzio All Natural Tropical Grill 10-Minute Marinade

163. Vidalia sweet onion relish

164. The Ginger People Sweet Ginger Chili Dipping & Cooking Sauce

165. Robert Rothschild Roasted Red Pepper & Onion Dip & Relish

166. Festin Roasted Red Bell Pepper Sauce with Garlic & Herbs

167. Peanut butter transforms a basic white sauce into a versatile condiment that tastes good when spooned over cooked vegetables and veggie burger patties. It also makes a good dip for raw vegetables. In a small saucepan over low heat, whisk together 2 tablespoons corn oil and 2 tablespoons white flour. Stir for 3 to 4 minutes, taking care to keep the flour from sticking to the bottom of the pan. Slowly stir in 1 cup vegetable broth, followed by 1 tablespoon creamy peanut butter. Keep stirring until well blended. Simmer and stir the sauce for several minutes, until thickened and hot, but don't let it boil. Remove from the heat and serve. This makes a little more than a cup of sauce.

168. Steer clear of goopy cheese sauces on nachos. Plain, trans-fat-free tortilla chips and salsa are a delicious and much healthier choice.

169. You can't go wrong with marinara sauce on your pasta. Classic marinara sauce is made with tomatoes, olive oil, and

Italian herbs and spices. It is meatless, so there's no saturated fat or cholesterol. It is also trans-fat-free.

Bonus Tip: Work more vegetables into your diet. Grate or chop fresh vegetables such as broccoli, carrots, green peppers, mushrooms, onions, and kale, and blend them into marinara sauce while it is heating on the stove.

---

170. Surprise! **Fudge sauce on ice cream and other desserts is generally low in saturated fat and free of trans fat.** Unfortunately, it is high in calories, and the foods it's served on (ice cream, brownies, etc.) are rich in saturated fat and trans fat. Satisfy the urge with a scoop of the fudge sauce right out of the bottle, and stop there.

171. **Pesto sauce is an aromatic and healthy alternative to marinara sauce on pasta.** It is made by finely chopping and mixing together fresh basil leaves, pine nuts (also known as pignolis), olive oil, garlic, and salt. Pesto sauce is a classic and is perfect when tossed with angel-hair pasta or fettuccine. You can also

172. Stir a little into salad dressing.

173. Spread it on a sandwich or Italian bread rounds.

174. Blend some into nonfat plain yogurt for a dip.

175. Mix some into cooked rice or couscous.

176. **Make a refreshing and flavorful accompaniment to curried dishes** by mixing equal parts of chutney and plain nonfat yogurt.

Bonus Tip: If you have never tried chutney, make a point to pick some up and experiment with it. Chutneys are sweet and spicy. They go well on sandwiches and can be used as a relish or an ingredient in dips and sauces. Chutneys are typically associated with Indian food, but they're used throughout Southeast Asia. In the United States Major Grey's mango chutney is the most familiar brand sold in supermarkets.

---

177. Create your own simple sauces to use over side dishes and entrees or to double as dips and sandwich spreads. Experiment with combinations of fruits and vegetables, processed until smooth in a blender or food processor. Try roasted red bell peppers and sun-dried tomatoes, or onions, roasted red bell peppers, garlic, chopped fresh tomatoes, and olive oil.

178. Make your own barbecue sauce by mixing equal parts of molasses, soy sauce, and ketchup. It is easy to do and means one less bottle to compete for space in your refrigerator.

179. Salsa is not only a good dip for chips but also makes a tasty and healthy sauce on casseroles, veggie burger patties, beans and rice, and baked potatoes.

180. Make your own fresh salsa at home. In a food processor or blender, combine 2 tablespoons fresh lime juice, 2 cloves garlic, 1 small sweet onion, 4 ounces canned green chilies (no need to drain), ¼ teaspoon ground cumin, and ¼ teaspoon salt. Process until finely chopped. Add this mixture to 2½ cups chopped fresh tomatoes and chill for two hours before serving. Optional ways to spice it up include adding chopped cilantro to taste, substituting lemon juice for lime juice, or adding a chopped fresh avocado.

181. For another variation, add salsa to plain nonfat yogurt, soy mayonnaise, or a mixture of the two for a creamy salsa sauce.

Chapter 9

Get the Trans Fat Out
of Entrees and Side Dishes

Dietary advice in general—and detailed advice about how to avoid trans fat—often leaves people feeling depressed about their food choices. No fries. No biscuits. No margarine. No fun.

An e-mail I received from a reader of my weekly newspaper column, in which I discussed the need for many of us to cut back on cheese (because of its saturated fat content), says it well: "When I saw Thursday's screed against cheese, I thought, 'What's next?' Is my diet to be reduced to steamed rutabagas and tofu? It seems that each week a different (and yummy) food hits the 'limited,' 'very limited,' or 'no-no' list. The end result is I no longer listen."

While there are rarely absolute yes and no foods, it is fair to say that some foods—especially in the amounts typically eaten by most Americans—are clearly better for you than others. Orange juice is better than a soft drink. Bananas are better than a candy bar. Olive oil is better than butter or margarine. And cheese, like any foods that contain trans fat and saturated fat, is something most of us need to limit in order to preserve our health.

But discussions about how to eat well should focus not only on foods you should limit but also the flip side: foods to eat in greater quantities. The trouble is, all that many people hear is the negative message: what *not* to eat. They have a harder time envisioning what they *can* eat. One of the hurdles of understanding dietary advice is integrating the dos as well as the don'ts into a mental vision of the total diet. In this chapter, therefore, I'll try to help you do just that.

By paying attention to the two primary goals I've been focusing on all along in this book—eating *fewer* unhealthy foods and *more* healthy foods—we can accomplish our goals of getting the trans fat out of entrees and side dishes. Because they're linked, my recommendations will also encourage you to eat less saturated fat in these big items that you eat every day.

In the case of entrees and sides, following my advice may require you to rethink your vision of what a meal looks like. That's because, in a good diet that supports health, the foods most of us think of as side dishes trade places with the foods we tend to think of as the focal point of the meal. For instance, I'll encourage you to double and triple your servings of salad, broccoli, sweet potatoes, and rice, and shrink the amount of meat and cheese you eat—to use them as condiments or even push them off your plate entirely. This does leave plenty to eat—far more than rutabagas and tofu! But it might also require you to adopt a new mindset about food.

A few years back I interviewed health guru Jack LaLanne, still mentally and physically fit and active at nearly ninety years of age. His approach to eating stuck with me: "Figure out what's good for you, then create a liking for it," he said. It is advice worth taking.

Great Grains

182. Whole grains, such as wheat, rice, barley, millet, and oats, can be used as the foundation of many casseroles and main-dish pilafs or as side dishes alone or mixed with vegetables and other ingredients.

183. Grains are free of trans fat and saturated fat, and are valuable sources of protein, B vitamins, fiber, and minerals. They vary in their nutritional content but are generally safe and healthy. They vary in flavor, too.

> Bonus Tip: For a summary of whole-grain cooking and storage instructions, go online to Whole Foods Market at www.wholefoodsmarket.com/recipes/tips_grains.html.

184. Rice is one of the least allergenic foods. It is not only the nutritious foundation of many healthy main dishes but is also very unlikely to present a problem to you, your family, or dinner guests. That is why rice cereal is a first baby food.

185. Rice eaters have better diets. That's the conclusion of an Iowa State University researcher who analyzed government data on American dietary intakes. Funded by the rice industry, the study found that people who eat rice are slimmer and have diets more in line with the 2005 Dietary Guidelines. Rice eaters' diets contain less added fat and sugar, and include more grains, vegetables, and fruits. That is how eating more rice also helps you get the trans fat out!

186. Countless great dishes use rice. Try making Spanish paella (a seasoned one-dish meal that combines rice with cooked vegetables and often small pieces of shrimp or scallops), jambalaya, Creole red beans and rice, Cuban black beans and rice, stir-fried vegetables and rice, or chili served over rice.

187. Use different types of rice in different dishes.

188. *Long grain.* The kernels are several times longer than their width. The steamed rice is light and fluffy because kernels stay separate. This is the type you're most likely to have at home in your pantry.

189. *Medium grain.* The kernels are a little shorter and moister, so they stick together a bit.

190. *Short grain.* Kernels are moist and rounded and clump together easily.

191. *Aromatic.* Popular varieties are jasmine and basmati, which have a nutty flavor and fragrance. Steamed basmati rice is light, fluffy, and long-grained. It is often served with Indian food. Jasmine rice is moister, so kernels stick together. You may have eaten it in Thai restaurants.

192. *Arborio.* A medium-grain rice that is creamy in texture when cooked. It is used to make an Italian dish called risotto.

Bonus Tip: Despite the differences in cooking properties and, in some cases, flavor, the different types of rice are similar in nutritional value.

---

193. Consider how the rice you use is processed. Brown rice is best. Only the outer hull is removed, leaving the bran layers that contain fiber and B vitamins. White rice has the hull removed and the bran layers milled or polished, leaving the grain white in color. It is still nutritious but less so than brown rice. Parboiled rice has been processed with steam to create firmer kernels that stay separated when cooked, making fluffier rice. Precooked rice has been cooked and dehydrated so that cooking time at home is greatly reduced.

194. If you buy boxes or bags of seasoned rice mixtures, read the nutrition facts labels and compare the sodium contents of different brands. Go for the lowest you can find. Better yet, buy plain rice and add your own herbs and low-sodium spices.

Bonus Tip: Trans fat alert! If a packaged mix calls for added margarine or butter, use vegetable oil instead.

---

195. Cooking rice is easy. Add 1 cup brown rice to 2 cups boiling water, reduce the heat to low, and cook with the lid on the pot for about 50 minutes, or until all the water is absorbed.

196. Consider purchasing a rice cooker. They resemble slow cookers and make perfectly steamed fluffy rice without requiring stove top supervision. Add water and rice, set the timer, and walk away. The cooker keeps rice hot until you're ready to eat it.

197. Make more than you need. You can store leftover rice in an airtight container for several days in the refrigerator or for months in the freezer and then use it later in another dish.

198. One type of rice can usually be substituted for another in recipes. The exception is the creamy arborio rice.

199. For a change of pace, consider cooking with some ancient grains familiar in other parts of the world where they have been used for centuries. Here are two grains worth a trip to a natural foods store to buy.

200. *Amaranth* has been eaten for generations in Central and South America and was a staple of the Aztecs. Amaranth isn't a true cereal grain; the "grains" are actually fruits of plants rather than grasses. The plant is broad-leafed, producing thousands of little seeds about the size of poppy seeds. These are sold in natural foods stores as a whole grain (or intact grain) or flour, and you'll see amaranth listed as an ingredient in breakfast cereals and crackers. Steamed, it's a side dish or hot cereal. It can also be used in casseroles, baked goods, and pancakes, and it can even be popped like popcorn. It has a strong, spicy, nutty flavor that may taste better in some recipes than others, and it can be blended with other grains.

201. *Quinoa* (KEEN-wah) is a high-protein grain that was eaten by the Incas in Peru and is popular today around the world because of its good taste and nutritional value. Quinoa grains (also technically the fruit of the plant) are tiny and flat, and range in color from white or yellow to dark brown. Unwashed quinoa is coated with saponin, a substance that lathers when wet and is mildly toxic. Quinoa purchased in packages is usually prewashed, but it doesn't hurt to rinse it again before using. Cook it and use it like rice in casseroles, pilaf, salads, or as a side dish with cooked vegetables.

202. Packaged foods made with whole grains are less likely to contain trans fat than foods with refined grains such as white flour. How do you know a whole grain when you see one? The easiest way is to read the food label and look for one word: *whole.* Look for whole wheat, whole rye, whole oats, and so on. Ingredients are listed in order of their predominance in the product. If whole wheat is the first ingredient listed, it probably makes up at least half of that product.

> Bonus Tip: Wheat flour is refined white flour. If it were whole, it would say so. Take bread, for example. Just because it's brown doesn't mean it is made from whole wheat. It could be caramel coloring. Always check the label!

203. Take the flavor up a notch! **Try using vegetable broth in place of water** when you cook grains.

204. Whole-grain pasta is another good base for trans-fat-free healthy entrees. Many supermarkets carry Hodgson Mills whole wheat pasta, and many other brands are available at natural foods stores. As with other whole-grain products, whole wheat pasta has more flavor and a heavier texture than white pasta. Do be aware that it has a tendency to become gummy if it is overcooked. It grows on you, though, as people who have switched from white to whole wheat bread already know.

205. Try some great new dishes using whole wheat pasta, such as a pesto pasta tossed with sun-dried tomatoes, artichoke hearts, and black olives.

206. Toss pasta with wilted greens, olive oil, chopped walnuts, and a sprinkling of Parmesan cheese.

207. Pasta with chopped broccoli, mushrooms, carrots, and onions is delicious.

208. You might also try pasta with fresh chopped tomatoes, low-fat shredded mozzarella cheese, chopped walnuts, capers, and fresh basil.

209. You can also mix in marinara sauce with soy burger crumbles (which has less saturated fat than sauce made with ground beef).

Better with Beans

210. Homemade entrees made with beans, peas, and lentils are quick and easy to make. They're free of trans fat and are super nutritious. Where else can you get as much protein and fiber—up to 16 grams of each in a cup—with virtually no saturated fat or cholesterol and substantial amounts of calcium, iron, and folate? Certainly not in meat! Beans are also low in sodium and rich in complex carbohydrates.

Bonus Tip: Beans are the perfect "prevention" food. The fiber load in beans—just one cup gives you about half of the fiber you need in a day—is associated with several health benefits such as:

Weight control. Beans are bulky but relatively low in calories, so they fill you up without filling you out.

Gastrointestinal health. Fiber-rich beans help prevent constipation, hemorrhoids, and diverticular disease.

Heart health. The soluble fiber in beans helps lower blood cholesterol levels. Eating beans regularly, especially when they displace high-fat meat or dairy products, helps reduce the risk of coronary artery disease.

Diabetes control. The soluble fiber in beans helps lower and stabilize blood sugar levels.

Cancer control. Diets high in beans are also associated with lower rates of some forms of cancer.

211. Beans come in many varieties. The kind I'm suggesting for entrees—legumes—are not to be confused with green beans and wax beans. Dry legumes grow in a pod and are oval shaped. Examples of these especially nutritious kinds of beans include pinto, black, navy, lima, kidney, and garbanzo. Unique heirloom varieties are also available at farmers' markets and through mail order.

212. Dried beans, especially darkly pigmented varieties, are also a rich source of the antioxidants commonly associated with deeply colored fruits and vegetables. Black beans in particular have high concentrations of flavonoids, a type of antioxidant associated with reduced rates of coronary artery disease, cancer, and aging. They contain more than ten times the antioxidant level per serving as oranges and about the same amount as grapes, apples, and cranberries.

213. If you're wondering what to make for dinner tonight, **try a black bean burrito.** I make a knockoff of the Flying

Mayan Burrito, a black bean burrito served at the Flying Burrito restaurant near my home in North Carolina. Seasoned black beans, mashed sweet potato, rice, and avocado are wrapped in a flour tortilla and topped with shredded lettuce, tomato, black olives, and salsa. I use nonfat plain yogurt instead of sour cream. It's trans-fat-free and delicious.

214. Canned, frozen, or flaked beans are quick and basically healthy. The most convenient way to buy dry beans is canned and precooked. I prefer organically grown canned beans. Remember to remove most of the salt added in the canning process by rinsing the canned beans with cold water in a colander before using. Some supermarkets also carry frozen lima beans and blackeyed peas; thaw and rinse them before use. Dehydrated pinto bean and black bean flakes are available in natural foods stores; add hot water and stir them.

215. An alternative to using canned beans or bean flakes is to buy dry beans and rehydrate them yourself. It takes time to cook with fresh dry beans, but they're low in sodium (unless you add it). You can speed up the process by using a pressure cooker. Otherwise, you'll have to prepare them slowly, the old-fashioned way. That involves soaking beans in water before cooking to soften them. Slow cookers are convenient for that purpose, too; the longer the beans cook, the softer they become.

216. Dry beans are a staple in healthy entrees around the world. Here are some delectable examples:

- American navy bean soup
- Italian pasta e fagioli (pasta with white beans)
- Middle Eastern hummus and falafel (made with garbanzo beans)
- Mexican refried beans

- Cuban black beans and rice
- Creole red beans and rice

217. If the thought of eating beans makes you think, "Beans, beans, the musical food," don't worry. **There are ways to eat beans without becoming a gastrointestinal mess.** When you add a lot of high-fiber foods to your diet, do it gradually and give it a little time. Your body adjusts to a higher fiber intake over time, and gas subsides. Be sure to drink plenty of fluids. Get moving, too. Physical activity causes gas to dissipate. And if worse comes to worst, there's always Beano, an over-the-counter gas reduction aid that you add to meals with "problem" foods. But, remember, it's true: Beans *are* good for the heart—and the rest of your body, too.

218. **Always remember to read food labels carefully.** Some packaged, seasoned bean mixtures sold in supermarkets contain partially hydrogenated oils.

219. **If you need recipes for healthy entrees you can make with beans,** there are two books I highly recommend: *Bean Banquets from Boston to Bombay* by Patricia Gregory (Woodbridge Press, 1983) and *Fabulous Beans* by Barb Bloomfield (Book Publishing Company, 1994).

220. It was mentioned in Chapter 8, but it bears repeating here: **Soup is a perfect entree because it is highly nutritious and low in calories.** Bean soups are the gold standard. Serve them for dinner at least once a week. Bean, lentil, and split pea soups are great choices because they're rich in fiber and protein. Serve them with some crusty bread and a tossed green salad to make a whole delicious meal.

221. **Lentils are as nutritious as dried beans and can take less time to cook.** Though they're sold dried in plastic bags like other legumes, don't let their appearance put you off; they really are much less time-consuming than other beans sold the same way. Lentils—small disk-shaped seeds from a bushy plant—are one of the world's oldest legumes. They've been on the menu for thousands of years in the Middle East, India, Eastern Africa, and the Mediterranean, and today they're grown and eaten throughout Europe, Canada, and the United States as well. Some of the foods you can order in ethnic restaurants today— Indian dal and curries, lentil soups, and stews—are largely unchanged from recipes used since the dawn of agriculture in countries such as Pakistan, Afghanistan, Iraq, Egypt, Greece, and Ethiopia. You can easily make these at home yourself.

222. **Most mainstream supermarkets carry brown lentils.** You'll find them near the dried beans and split peas. But there are dozens of different kinds of lentils ranging in color from greenish brown to orange, yellow, and red. I buy mine in large bags in Indian food markets. Check the phone book for ethnic food markets near you. If you haven't been inside one of these little markets, you'll be surprised at the variety of fruits, vegetables, and condiments stocked there that you don't see in mainstream stores.

Bonus Tip: If you buy more lentils than you need for one meal, store the remainder in an airtight container or jar at room temperature. Lentils keep for at least a year under these conditions. Be sure to rotate stock, though. If you buy a new bag of lentils before the old supply is used up, keep the fresh supply separate from the old. Older lentils are drier than fresh ones and take longer to cook.

---

223. **Lentil soup makes a good entree.** Top it with some chopped fresh onion and a sprig of parsley or stir in leftover cooked spinach. This simple recipe takes only ten minutes to fix and an hour to cook on the stove top.

Easy Lentil Soup

PREP TIME: 10 MINUTES

COOKING TIME: 1 HOUR

Yield: 8 servings

1¼ cups dried brown lentils
1 medium to large onion
1 teaspoon minced garlic
5 cups water
Salt and freshly ground black pepper to taste
2 tablespoons olive oil
One 16-ounce can stewed or crushed tomatoes
1 bay leaf

1. Rinse the lentils in a colander and chop the onion.
2. Combine in a large saucepan the lentils, onion, garlic, water, salt, pepper, and olive oil. Cover and cook over medium heat for about 15 minutes.
3. Stir in the tomatoes and bay leaf. Reduce the heat to low and simmer for 45 minutes, or until the lentils are tender. Serve hot.

224. You'll find **some easy delicious recipes for entrees made with lentils** in *The Meatless Gourmet: Easy Lowfat Favorites* by Bobbie Hinman (Prima Publishing, 1997), which you can order online.

225. Remember pressure cookers; they can help you produce a two-hour meal in ten minutes. They can reduce the cooking time of dried beans considerably. Refer to Chapter 5 for more about them. And remember, pressure cookers have gotten much more stable since the rickety contraptions in your mother's kitchen.

Holding It All Together

226. In savory dishes such as casseroles and meat loaves, you can reduce your overall trans fat/saturated fat/cholesterol quotient by replacing one whole egg with 2 to 3 tablespoons quick-cooking rolled oats or cooked oatmeal.

227. Or use 2 to 3 tablespoons mashed potatoes, mashed sweet potatoes, or instant potato flakes. They work as binders but are bland and don't interfere with other flavors.

228. Or use 2 to 3 tablespoons fine bread crumbs, cracker meal, or matzo meal. These items will keep for months stored in an airtight container in the pantry.

229. Or use 2 to 3 tablespoons flour. White, whole wheat—any kind will do.

230. Or use 2 to 3 tablespoons arrowroot starch, potato starch, cornstarch, or EnerG Egg Replacer mixed with 2 tablespoons water. They're flavorless and work well in most recipes.

231. Or use 2 to 3 tablespoons tomato paste. Since so little is used, the tomato flavor doesn't compete with other flavors in most entree recipes.

Soy Delicious

232. Soybeans are phytochemical factories; they contain plant chemicals that protect health. Soybeans are a rich source of isoflavones, including genistein and daidzein. They and other phytochemicals may be responsible for health benefits such as a lowered risk of some forms of cancer.

233. Packaged soy-based entrees such as vegetarian meat loaf and lasagna sold in natural foods stores are unlikely to contain partially hydrogenated oils and are trans-fat-free. The same is mainly true for those sold in mainstream supermarkets, but it's always a good practice to double-check nutrition labels just to be sure.

234. **Processed soy products come in many forms** and can be used to make an almost infinite number of healthy trans-fat-free entrees at home. Products such as burger crumbles, veggie burger patties, soy hotdogs, and soy sausage patties and bacon substitute can be used to make dozens of dishes. Here are some ideas:

> **235.** Meatless "meat" loaves and Swedish "meat" balls
>
> **236.** Burrito and taco fillings
>
> **237.** Pasta topped with "meaty" sauce
>
> **238.** "Beef" and bean chili
>
> **239.** Soy burgers and notdogs grilled outdoors
>
> **240.** Beans and franks
>
> **241.** Pizza topped with crumbled "sausage" and veggies
>
> **242.** Casseroles topped with "bacon," or "bacon" used in split pea soup or on a main-course spinach salad

243. **Textured vegetable protein (TVP)** is a soy product that can replace ground beef in recipes such as chili, spaghetti sauce, and sloppy joe sandwich filling (see the recipe on page 136). It is sold as burger crumbles in supermarkets in the freezer section or dried in small chunks or bits in bags, boxes, or in bulk at natural foods stores. It is also available by mail order at online stores such as The Mail Order Catalog at www.healthy-eating.com.

244. **Tofu is one of the best-known soy foods.** It is an odorless, flavorless block of soybean curd used in Asian stir-fries such as the Buddha's Delight served at Chinese restaurants. It is trans-fat-free. It can also radically reduce the saturated fat load of traditional cheese-laden entrees; for example, it can be crumbled and used in combination with or in place of ricotta cheese in Italian entrees (such as manicotti and lasagna).

> Bonus Tip: Freezing tofu and then thawing it causes it to develop a chewy texture that resembles that of meat.

245. Bookstores and the library offer many good books on cooking with soy foods. Here are a few of my favorites:

246. *Tofu Cookery*, revised edition, by Louise Hagler (Book Publishing Company, 1991). This oversized paperback book is a classic. The photos alone are worth the cost of the book.

247. *More Soy Cooking*, by Marie Oser (Wiley, 2000)

248. *The Complete Soy Cookbook*, by Paulette Williams (Macmillan, 1998)

249. Tempeh is an equally versatile and, in my opinion, tastier and more practical soy food that you should consider trying. Tempeh is easy to use, and like tofu, it picks up the flavors of foods it is cooked with. You can use it in place of meat in recipes for chili, soups, stews, sauces, and casseroles. It can be grilled and used as an entree or an ingredient in sandwich and burrito fillings. Tempeh is a rich source of protein and a good source of riboflavin, thiamin, niacin, calcium, iron, and zinc. It is low in saturated fat, is cholesterol- and trans-fat-free, and is full of beneficial phytochemicals. Some of my favorite ways to use tempeh include the following:

250. *As a sandwich filling.* Use it crumbled in place of beef in recipes for sloppy Joes, mock chicken salad, or even to make barbecue. Strips can also be barbecued or grilled and served in TLTs (tempeh, lettuce, and tomato sandwiches) on toasted whole-grain bread.

251. *In burritos, tacos, and fajitas.* Cut it into strips and grill it. Delicious!

252. *In shish kebab.* Use grilled or marinated chunks of tempeh with vegetables on skewers, and serve with rice pilaf and pita pockets.

253. *In Asian-inspired dishes.* Panfry cubes of tempeh in soy-ginger sauce and serve with cooked greens and steamed rice.

254. To soften tempeh and make it easier to crumble, steam it for a few minutes in a steamer basket or over a pot of boiling water. Be sure to let it cool before handling. Tempeh used in recipes that call for slabs or strips doesn't usually require any special preparation first.

Bonus Tip: Some supermarkets carry tempeh, but you're most likely to find it in the refrigerated and frozen foods sections of natural foods stores. It is usually sold in 8-ounce vacuum-packed packages. Tempeh keeps for about a week in the refrigerator or several months in the freezer. I usually buy several packages at a time and keep them in the freezer until needed. You can thaw tempeh in the refrigerator overnight or in a couple of minutes in a microwave oven. Like meats and other high-protein foods, tempeh should not be left at room temperature for more than two hours.

---

255. For an introduction to cooking with tempeh, try *The Tempeh Cookbook,* by Dorothy Bates (Book Publishing Company, 1989). It's a skinny little paperback classic with a few color photographs and simple recipes.

256. Reduce the combined load of trans fat and saturated fat in cheesy entrees by incorporating soy-based cheese. Several types of soy cheese are available, including mozzarella, American, and cream cheese. You'll find the most variety at natural foods stores. Any variety can be used in place of regular cheese in recipes, although, like most nonfat dairy cheeses, soy cheese doesn't melt as well as full-fat dairy cheeses. Soy cheese works best when used as one of many ingredients in a recipe; for example, it's better used in lasagna than alone on a cracker.

Cheesy Solutions

257. **Lower the combined total of bad fat in many casseroles and other mixed dishes by cutting the fat from cheese.** You'll find the largest selection of cheese alternatives at natural foods stores, including soy- and nut-based versions of mozzarella, jack, cheddar, Parmesan, and cream cheese. Most cheese substitutes work best as an ingredient in a mixed dish rather than alone as an appetizer with crackers or in grilled cheese sandwiches where the difference in flavor may be more apparent.

258. **Try this trans-fat-free and saturated-fat-free homemade cheese substitute** created by Joanne Stepaniak, author of *The Ultimate Uncheese Cookbook* (Book Publishing Company, 2003). It tastes great, and you can eat it on crackers and sandwiches, spread it on veggie burgers to make healthy "cheeseburgers," or use it in almost any recipe that calls for cheddar or American-style cheese.

Gee Whiz Spread

Yield: 2 cups

2 cups (one 15- or 16-ounce can) drained cooked or canned white beans

½ cup roasted red pepper (skin and seeds removed) or pimiento pieces

6 to 8 tablespoons nutritional yeast flakes (found in natural
   foods stores)
3 tablespoons fresh lemon juice
2 to 3 tablespoons sesame tahini or cashew butter
½ teaspoon prepared yellow mustard
½ teaspoon salt
¼ teaspoon each garlic and onion powder

Place all the ingredients in a food processor and process until
completely smooth and evenly colored (this may take several
minutes). Stop the processor and scrape down the sides of the
bowl as necessary during processing. Chill thoroughly before
serving. Keeps five to seven days in the refrigerator.

VARIATIONS: In place of the red peppers, use ½ cup carrots,
cooked and chopped, or ¾ teaspoon paprika, or 2 tablespoons
unsalted tomato paste.

For an "aged cheddar" flavor, add 1 to 2 teaspoons light or
chickpea miso.

Bonus Tip: Soy- and nut-based cheeses melt better than
most nonfat dairy cheeses (though not as well as full-fat
dairy cheeses). That's because soy- and nut-based
cheeses are relatively high in vegetable fat, which im-
proves meltability.

---

259. Make a nondairy substitute for ricotta cheese or cottage
cheese by mashing a chunk of tofu and blending it with a few
teaspoons of lemon juice. Use it in place of or in combination
with the ricotta or cottage cheese in recipes for Italian stuffed
shells, lasagna, casseroles, and other mixed dishes.

260. Nutritional yeast has a savory cheesy flavor that makes
it a good substitute for Parmesan cheese on casseroles and

pasta. You can also use it on salads, baked potatoes, and popcorn. You'll find it at natural foods stores.

261. For the kids in your life, **try this healthy version of macaroni and cheese,** also from Joanne Stepaniak's *The Ultimate Uncheese Cookbook.* According to Joanne, "This recipe is reminiscent of 'cafeteria-style' macaroni and cheese—it has a dry rather than creamy consistency, because as it bakes, the 'cheese' forms tiny curds around the pasta. Kids of all ages will adore it."

Baked Macaroni & Cheez

Yield: 8 servings

*2 tablespoons olive or organic canola or safflower oil plus more
    for oiling a dish*
1 large onion, finely chopped
*4 cups (16 ounces) dry macaroni or other tube pasta (such as
    penne or ziti)*
2 cups water
*½ cup roasted red pepper (skin and seeds removed) or pimiento
    pieces*
½ cup raw cashews or ⅓ cup cashew butter
⅓ cup fresh lemon juice
⅓ cup nutritional yeast flakes
¼ cup white wine
2 teaspoons onion powder
2 teaspoons garlic powder
1 teaspoon salt

1. Preheat the oven to 350 degrees. Oil a 3-quart casserole dish or mist it with nonstick cooking spray and set aside. (Alternatively, use a nonstick casserole dish.)

2. Heat the oil in a large saucepan. When hot, add the onion and sauté until tender and lightly browned, about 15 to 20 minutes.

3. Meanwhile, cook the macaroni according to package directions. Drain well and stir into the cooked onions. Mix well.

4. Combine the remaining ingredients in a blender and process for several minutes, until completely smooth. Stir into the macaroni and onions, and then spoon into the prepared casserole dish.

5. Bake, uncovered, for 25 to 35 minutes. Serve at once.

Ethnic Entrees

262. **Foods from other cultures offer a wide range of trans-fat-free meal options.** In contrast to the American meat-and-potatoes tradition, many other cultures have traditionally eaten foods that are plant-based and lower in saturated fat, and most other cultures are less dependent on packaged ingredients that are likely to contain trans fats. Healthy examples include Indian curried vegetables, Chinese stir-fry, Italian pasta e fagioli (pasta with beans), and Cuban black beans and rice. Eating more ethnic entrees also increases the pleasure of good food because there are more choices and more variation in flavors, colors, and aromas.

263. **If you have kids, it's a good idea to expose them to healthy trans-fat-free foods by offering them more unfamiliar ethnic foods.** In our home we often serve a new food alongside something familiar, with little fanfare. Just set it out and let them try it if they want to. Remember, kids learn by imitation, so let them see you eating and enjoying it.

264. **As an introduction to cuisines of other cultures, try ordering foods at ethnic restaurants.** (There will be more on this topic in Chapter 12.) It's a good way to find out what you like, and foods you eat out can serve as models for dishes you try making at home. Ditto for prepared foods from the supermarket. Natural foods stores often have good prices on Indian and Asian frozen entrees, all trans-fat-free, and if you especially like one, you can try to create it in your kitchen.

265. A good resource for ethnic recipes you can make easily and quickly at home is *The Meatless Gourmet: Favorite Recipes from Around the World* by Bonnie Hinman (Prima Publishing, 1995). Here's a recipe you can try that has zero trans fat and zero saturated fat.

Sweet 'n' Sour Chickpea Stew

Yield: eight 1½-cup servings

2 teaspoons vegetable oil
2 medium onions, sliced
Two 1-pound cans salt-free (or regular) tomatoes, chopped and undrained
One 19-ounce can chickpeas, rinsed and drained, or 2¼ cups cooked beans
1 cup water
½ cup molasses
½ cup vinegar
½ cup raisins
1 cup carrots, sliced crosswise into ½-inch chunks
2 large potatoes (1¼ pounds total), unpeeled and cut into ½-inch chunks
½ medium cabbage, coarsely chopped (about 4 cups)
1 teaspoon celery salt
¾ teaspoon ground ginger
¼ teaspoon pepper

1. Heat the oil in a large soup pot over medium heat. Add the onions, separating them into rings. Cook for 5 minutes, stir-

ring frequently and adding small amounts of water, a few tablespoons at a time, to prevent sticking.

2. Add the remaining ingredients and bring to a boil, stirring frequently.

3. Reduce the heat to medium-low, cover, and simmer for 40 minutes, or until the vegetables are tender.

266. I also like *Vegetarian Planet,* by Didi Emmons (Harvard Common Press, 1997), a James Beard Foundation Award for Excellence nominee. Here is one of my favorites from this book, a recipe with Italian origins.

Ziti with Acorn Squash and Roasted Garlic

Yield: 4 servings

1 acorn squash
15 large garlic cloves, peeled
6 tablespoons olive oil
1 pound dried ziti tubes or penne
⅓ cup white wine
½ teaspoon salt, or to taste
Freshly ground black pepper to taste
⅔ cup grated Parmesan cheese, plus more for
*   garnish*
¼ cup chopped walnuts, lightly toasted

1. Preheat the oven to 375 degrees. Cut the acorn squash in half, remove the seeds, and place the halves on a baking sheet, cut side down. Bake the squash for 1 hour, or until the flesh is soft. Let the squash cool, then spoon out the flesh from the shells and chop it fine.

2. About 30 minutes after the squash has begun baking, roast the garlic: Toss together the oil and garlic, and place them in

(continued)

an ovenproof dish. Bake the garlic, uncovered, alongside the squash for 30 minutes, or until the garlic is lightly golden.

3. Bring a large pot of salted water to a boil and cook the ziti until it is just tender. Drain it, reserving ¾ cup drained pasta water.

4. While the pasta cooks, spoon the roasted garlic with its oil into a large skillet. Add the wine and reserved pasta water, and bring the mixture to a boil. Let it boil for about 2 minutes. Add the chopped squash flesh and boil 3 minutes more. Take the skillet off the heat.

5. Add the ziti to the sauce and stir well. Add the salt, pepper, and Parmesan, and toss. Divide the pasta among four plates, sprinkle the walnuts over, and serve along with additional Parmesan.

NOTE: To lower the saturated fat content from 2.5 grams per serving to about 1 gram per serving, reduce the Parmesan cheese from ⅔ cup to ⅓ cup.

267. If you want to branch out and eat more ethnic foods but are not super daring, start with foods you think you'll like. If you like baked beans or pinto beans, try Indian dal (lentil soup), a Caribbean bean bake, or an Ethiopian lentil or bean stew.

268. The Mediterranean diet rules. It is naturally low in trans fat because it emphasizes fresh foods cooked in olive oil. The Mediterranean diet represents a cultural approach to food and lifestyle that dates back to antiquity. It includes influences from all of the coastal Mediterranean, including Portugal; the southern regions of Italy, Spain, and France; Turkey, Greece, and the western regions of Lebanon and Israel; and the northern areas of Egypt, Libya, Algeria, and Morocco. That makes for a wonderful diversity of dishes based on fresh seasonal foods that are locally grown and minimally processed. Here are just a few examples of the kinds of foods in the Mediterranean diet.

269. Vegetable stew made with eggplant, potatoes, zucchini, okra, and greens cooked in olive oil, garlic, onions, and herbs

270. Hearty lentil or fava bean soup

271. Eggplant pilaf or couscous with vegetables and fish

272. Pasta with beans or marinara sauce

273. Grape leaves, stuffed with rice, nuts, and vegetables

274. Grilled vegetable kebabs with steamed rice

275. Risotto with vegetables and seafood

Ready-made Entrees and Other Packaged Foods

276. Be a label reader first and foremost. This suggestion is repeated because it is so very important. If it is not fresh and made from scratch at home, it is a potential source of trans fat.

277. Don't be fooled by package labels that cry, "Trans-fat-free!" If it's high in saturated fat, it's still a poor choice. Read labels and add the grams of both trans fat and saturated fat to get the total amount of bad fat in a product. Aim for as little bad fat as possible.

278. If the amounts of trans fat or saturated fat on food packages seem low, check the serving size before digging in. If the food company has given information for unrealistically small serving sizes, you may eat two or three servings at a sitting and take in more fat that you planned.

279. Look for reduced-fat products. They tend to be lower in saturated fat and trans fat than their regular counterparts.

280. Be alert for packaged foods that don't list trans fat on the food label. Even though the new labeling regulations requiring trans fat to be listed went into effect in January 2006, some food companies persuaded the Food and Drug Administration to give them an extension. So items that don't have trans fat listed on the label at all are not necessarily trans-fat-free. You'll need to read the ingredient list to see if the product contains partially hydrogenated vegetable oil.

281. Dilute the trans fat or saturated fat in a frozen entree by splitting it into two servings. Round out your meal with additional servings of fresh vegetables, bread, and fruit.

Vegetables Side and Center

282. Substantially increasing your portions of vegetable side dishes is healthy in many ways; they're good for you, and you'll eat less of a main course that might involve meats or cheeses and other fatty foods. Eat heaping helpings of cooked fresh vegetables and shrink your entree portions. Another way to look at it: Pull the sides to the center and push the entree to the side.

283. Any side dish can be served as a main dish, and any entree can be a side dish. It is really just a matter of how you think about it and present it.

284. Take a chance on something new. Remember that you won't like *everything* you try, but if you try unfamiliar foods, you'll find some new favorites. Spend extra time in the produce aisle at the supermarket and try vegetables that are new to you. For example, kohlrabi, a nutritious root vegetable, is familiar to many Europeans but is less well known to most Americans.

285. Mix mashed bananas into refried beans, a good side dish or burrito filling.

286. Green or yellow plantains can be eaten as a cooked vegetable. Slice them and panfry them in olive oil, or mash them and serve them like mashed potatoes. Plantains are a close relative of the banana, but they are larger and more angular and are healthier for you than potatoes. Find them in supermarkets near the tropical fruits and bananas.

287. If you're looking for recipes for uncommon but delicious trans-fat-free side dishes, try Mollie Katzen's *Vegetable Heaven* (Hyperion, 1997).

288. In the summertime, take advantage of an abundance of backyard or produce-stand tomatoes and use them to make interesting side dishes. Here are some ideas:

289. Brush tomato halves with olive oil, top them with wheat germ or bread crumbs, and broil them in the oven.

290. Stuff tomato halves with couscous or rice pilaf and serve them as a side dish or an entree with other cooked vegetables.

291. Sauté fresh tomato pieces or cherry tomatoes in olive oil with other vegetables and season with oregano, basil, tarragon, or other herbs and spices.

292. Keep your levels of bad fats down by skipping the cheese sauce on the broccoli. Eat broccoli brushed with olive oil and a squirt of fresh lemon juice instead. Likewise, use nonfat yogurt or salsa on your baked potato instead of sour cream.

293. Grow to love fresh greens. Greens are leafy, headless relatives of the cabbage family: collards, mustard greens, and kale. They're superrich sources of calcium; iron; potassium; vitamins A, C, and E; folic acid; and fiber—and they don't contain a speck of trans fat or saturated fat. Add vinegar or hot sauce as they do in the South, but leave out the artery-clogging bacon grease. And here are some other trans-fat-free ways to eat greens:

294. In *The Vegetarian Soul Food Cookbook* (Epiphany Books, 2001), authors Imar Hutchins and Dawn Marie Daniels recommend seasoning mustard greens with sesame oil, balsamic vinegar, vegetable bouillon, red onion, and a little salt and pepper.

295. Also from Imar and Dawn's book, **give your collards "that hamhock taste that makes soul food distinctive"** by using liquid smoke seasoning along with a little olive oil, vegetable bouillon, vinegar, onion, and salt and pepper.

296. Add greens to other cooked vegetable mixtures. You can use up leftover cooked greens by tossing them with curried couscous and garbanzo beans.

297. **Use cooked greens in place of cabbage leaves** for making cabbage rolls or wrapping other rice, bean, or vegetable mixtures.

298. Sauté mixed greens (any combination of collards, mustards, or kale) with garlic, onions, and olive oil, and serve with cooked black-eyed peas and corn bread.

Bonus Tip: If you buy fresh greens, use them as soon as possible. To store, wrap the leaves in damp paper or cloth towels and place them in an open plastic bag or in the vegetable compartment of the refrigerator. They'll keep for up to a few days but will begin to yellow and go limp soon after. Wash fresh greens by swishing them around in a bowl or sink full of water to remove any dirt or grit. Greens with curly, rippled leaves may need to be rinsed two or three times to remove all the dirt. Give them a final rinse under the faucet and set them aside in a colander to drain or pat dry with a towel.

---

299. If you can't find fresh greens, frozen greens are just as good, nutritionally speaking.

300. Another trans-fat-free superfood to include on your menu as often as you can is the sweet potato. Sweet potatoes are rich in fiber, potassium, and vitamins A and C. Try baked sweet potatoes topped with nonfat cottage cheese and cinnamon.

301. You can also try them topped with crushed pineapple and a squeeze of fresh lime juice.

302. They're also good baked and wrapped in aluminum foil, and you can take them to school or the office.

303. Try them boiled, mashed, and mixed with a little pure maple syrup, cinnamon, and raisins.

304. Make candied sweet potatoes mixed with stewed apple slices.

305. Mashed white potatoes go well with almost any entree, and they're much better tasting and just as simple to make from scratch as they are from a packaged mix. Plain mashed potatoes are great, but for a change of pace, try them in the following varieties:

306. Mixed half and half with mashed sweet potatoes, along with nutmeg, salt, and pepper

307. Mixed with olive oil and minced garlic

308. Mixed with caramelized onion, salt, and pepper

309. Steaming vegetables in a covered pot or in a small amount of water in a microwave oven will preserve their nutrients. Vitamin C, for example, is destroyed by long exposure to heat, and other vitamins and minerals leach out into cooking water. By cooking with minimal water for as little time as possible, you can minimize loss of nutrients.

310. A simple side may be all you need. In fact, a complicated entree such as a layered casserole or something with multiple ingredients—stews or a black bean and sweet potato burrito—may lose some of its appeal if paired with another dish that contains multiple ingredients. Those sorts of dishes are best served with little more than a side of steamed broccoli or an ear of corn.

311. French fries, especially from fast-food restaurants, are frequently full of trans fat, but you can make your own fries at home from scratch in minutes. No need for precise measurements for this one. Preheat the oven to 350 degrees. Coat a baking sheet with vegetable oil spray or olive oil. Wash as many white potatoes as you wish. Leaving the peels on, cut the potatoes into wedges—as thin or as thick as you like. Place them in a mixing bowl and sprinkle them with several shakes each of garlic powder, oregano, cayenne pepper, and paprika. Toss to coat. Spread the potatoes on the baking sheet and brush the tops with olive oil. Bake for 40 minutes, or until the potatoes are soft. Eat them as is or dip in ketchup, salsa, or malt vinegar. Leftovers are great reheated.

312. Vegetable kebabs cooked on a grill are a festive and healthy addition to nearly any meal. Use a wooden skewer and assemble your kebabs using whole button mushrooms, cherry tomatoes, potato chunks, onion wedges, green pepper, and pineapple. Brush with olive oil and roast until the potatoes and onions are softened and the other ingredients are hot.

313. Use the vegetables you have. If you don't have an outdoor grill, roasted vegetables can be made by broiling them in a conventional oven.

314. Roasted root vegetables are another nutritious side dish, one that is especially nice when the weather turns crisp and cool. No measuring with this one, either. Peel and cut the following into 1-inch pieces or wedges: carrots, turnips, beets, parsnips, onions, and potatoes. Toss them with olive oil, minced garlic, rosemary, and salt and pepper to taste. Arrange the vegetables in one layer in an oiled dish or baking sheet and do not cover. Roast in a 350-degree oven for an hour or until tender. Remove the vegetables from the oven, toss them with several splashes of balsamic vinegar, and serve.

315. Fresh lemons and limes are indispensable and deserve a standing spot on your grocery list. Keep them handy to squeeze onto almost anything to give it a no-sodium, no-trans-fat zing.

316. Don't be afraid to experiment with new combinations of fruits, grains, vegetables, herbs, and spices. For inspiration, take some ideas from side-by-side dishes in Mollie Katzen's *Vegetable Heaven,* including these:

317. Roasted beans with garlic and olives

318. Soft lentils with roasted tomatoes and caramelized onions

319. Black beans in mango sauce

320. White beans with olive oil, garlic, and herbs

321. Wild rice pilaf with oranges and cherries

322. Spiced pineapple pilaf

323. Couscous with touches of orange, dill, and pistachio

324. Sizzling long beans with garlic and chilies

325. Green beans and tofu in crunchy Thai peanut sauce

326. Bitter greens with sweet onions and sour cherries

327. Sesame carrots on a bed of soft carrots

328. Cauliflower in tomato curry

329. Asparagus in warm tarragon-pecan vinaigrette

They are all trans-fat-free. Hungry yet?

Chapter 10

Get the Trans Fat Out of Snacks, Appetizers, and Sandwiches

Your intention is to eat better and lose a few pounds . . . and then the crackers start calling from the cupboard or someone passes around a cheese tray. Sandwiches, snacks, and appetizers are light meals and nibbles that people often eat on the run or as little extras between meals. They creep into most of our diets from time to time, if not daily, and they merit some attention.

The "quick and small" nature of these foods tends to lead to impulsive eating, and these foods can be rich in trans fat and saturated fat. Highly processed convenience foods—such as snack chips and commercial cookies and crackers—as well as fast-food sandwiches, hors d'oeuvres made with puff pastry, croissants, cheese, and other ingredients are loaded with bad fats. This chapter will help you identify the main culprits and will also help you find some satisfying and practical alternatives. (We'll cover fast food and sweet treats in Chapters 11 and 12.)

Whether we're noshing on healthy foods or junk, most of us would be better off eating less food altogether. Since the majority of us are overweight or trying to head off a weight problem, it would be beneficial to avoid excessive eating in the first place. There are some very effective steps you can take to lessen the likelihood of snacking and nibbling on foods you don't need between meals. Some simple strategies can short-circuit a binge or redirect your attention to nutritious lower-calorie foods.

The urge to snack is often caused by one of two things:

1. *A cue in the environment.* You could have a conditioned response to a certain time of day, the presence of a particular person, the act of watching TV or working at the computer, or the presence of an emotional state such as anger, frustration, or anxiety. You may be linking one of these conditions in your mind with "time to eat."

2. *Excessive hunger.* In this case, physiology weakens your resolve. Hungry people often make impulsive food choices and overeat.

What can you do to protect yourself from these hazards or minimize their impact? First, don't let yourself get too hungry. If you arrive home famished at the end of the day, you are more likely to gorge on whatever is quick and convenient, such as chips, cookies, or candy. Eat a well-timed snack in the late afternoon before you leave work, and you'll be better able to head off the kind of hunger that leads to binge eating and wait until dinner to eat.

Some people find that they need five or six small meals or snacks throughout the day to feel their best and to keep their appetite from getting out of control and leading them to binge. In that case, have a little something every two to three hours. A piece of fresh fruit, a bowl of cereal, a cup of soup, or a half sandwich (later we'll discuss what kind) are good choices.

The next step is to identify cues that trigger the urge to snack and recondition yourself not to follow them. A food diary can be an effective tool for helping you recognize problem areas. Record everything you eat and drink from the time you wake up until the time you go to bed. Use a notebook, index cards, or your computer—whatever works for you. Keep track of the details: how much you ate, what kind of food it was, the time, who was there, where you were, how you felt. The more detail, the better. Do it for several days, don't wait until the end of the day to write it down. Record each meal or snack immediately after finishing it.

Look for patterns. Do you have an irresistible urge to snack every evening in front of the television set? Then look for ways to reprogram that behavior. Either find something else to do during that time, such as going for a long walk, or busy yourself with something else, perhaps a household task, while watching your favorite show. Redirect yourself to an activity other than eating.

You have to snack and have light meals sometimes, of course. When you do, make sure that what you have on hand is what you want to eat. What should that be? Read on.

Sandwich Spreads and Fillers

330. Load up sandwiches with fresh fillers. Great choices include lettuce, tomato, and onion slices and chopped or shredded vegetables such as carrots and cucumbers.

331. Roasted red peppers add heft and flavor to virtually any sandwich. I buy peppers bottled in olive oil and keep them on hand in the refrigerator. Try whole wheat toast smeared with pesto, a layer of roasted red pepper, and one wafer-thin slice of reduced-fat provolone cheese. It's incredibly tasty and trans-fat-free!

332. Greatly reduce cheese in your sandwiches. They jack up your combined total of trans fat plus saturated fat. Cheese rates as the number one source of saturated fat in the American diet.

333. Pay attention to the kind of bread you're using. Build sandwiches between slices of good whole-grain breads, whole wheat pita pockets, or hard rolls. Remember that national dietary recommendations now say at least half of all the breads and cereals we eat should be made from fiber- and nutrient-rich whole grains rather than refined white grains.

334. Add personality to sandwiches. Try using fat-free condiments such as honey mustard, Dijon mustard, chutney, apple butter, jam, honey, or salsa to make sandwiches delicious while still being good for you.

335. The healthiest sandwich fillers are free of trans fat and saturated fat, low in cholesterol and sodium, and high in fiber. Here are some of my favorites and a few that, while unusual, are delicious and a nice change of pace from the usual PB&J:

336. Hummus and grated carrots in a pita pocket

337. Baby spinach leaves; grated carrots, onions, and mushrooms; tomato slices; sunflower seeds; and creamy Italian dressing in a pita pocket

338. Almond butter and pear slices on whole wheat bread

339. Peanut butter and banana on cinnamon raisin bread

340. Peanut butter and apple slices on sourdough bread

341. Cashew butter with peach slices

342. Almond butter topped with thinly sliced Granny Smith apple

343. A cooked veggie burger pattie with mustard and ketchup

344. Peanut butter mixed with chopped bell peppers and green onions

345. Avocado mashed with grated carrots and a little salsa with one slice of nonfat cheese

346. Sliced backyard tomatoes and yellow mustard on whole wheat toast

347. Hummus and tomato slices grilled with trans-fat-free margarine on multigrain bread

348. Sliced tomatoes with fresh basil leaves and one thin slice of fat-free cheese on whole-grain toast

349. Baked beans on whole wheat toast (This was mentioned in an earlier chapter, but it's so good that it merits a reminder!)

350. Leftover black bean dip, heated, and grated carrots rolled in a whole wheat flour tortilla

351. Vary the bread to give sandwiches more character. Peanut butter mixed with honey and mashed banana tastes great on a cinnamon raisin bagel or a wheat or spinach flour tortilla. Use whole wheat hotdog or hoagie rolls to make a sub sandwich using nonfat or very low fat cheese, lettuce, tomato slices, green pepper rings, sliced black olives, and ground black pepper. Try a PB&J made with banana bread.

352. Use tofu in place of egg in traditional egg salad recipes and replace regular mayo with soy mayonnaise. Try making this filling, which is good in sandwiches or stuffed into a scooped-out tomato half: In a medium bowl, mash one 8- or 10-ounce container of silken firm tofu and stir in 1 tablespoon yellow mustard, ½ teaspoon paprika, 2 stalks of celery, minced, ¼ cup pickle relish, ¼ teaspoon black pepper, 2 green onions, and ½ cup soy mayonnaise. Mix well and chill. Makes four ⅓-cup servings.

353. Blend peanut butter or almond butter with a little honey and/or chopped dried fruit pieces for a sandwich filling or for a spread on toast or crackers.

354. This recipe for a sloppy joe sandwich filling is from one of my favorite cookbooks, *The Peaceful Palate,* by Jennifer Raymond (Heart and Soul Publications, 1996). It contains no trans fat, saturated fat, or cholesterol.

Yield: 4 servings

1½ cups water
1 large onion, finely chopped
1 bell pepper, finely diced
1 cup textured vegetable protein (found at natural foods stores)
One 15-ounce can tomato sauce
1 tablespoon sugar or other sweetener
1 teaspoon chili powder
1 teaspoon garlic powder or granules
2 tablespoons cider vinegar
1 tablespoon soy sauce
1 teaspoon stone-ground mustard or Dijon mustard
4 whole wheat burger buns

1. Heat ½ cup water in a large pot, then add the onion and bell pepper. Cook until the onion is soft, about 5 minutes. Add the remaining 1 cup water, the textured vegetable protein, tomato sauce, sugar, chili powder, garlic powder, cider vinegar, soy sauce, and mustard. Cook over medium heat, stirring frequently, for 10 minutes.

2. Split the buns and warm them in a toaster. Top with a serving of sauce.

355. Enjoy a guilt-free (and delicious) BLT sandwich using lettuce, tomato, soy mayonnaise, and soy-based "bacon" strips on whole wheat toast. Try Lightlife Fakin' Bacon Strips or Morningstar Farms Veggie Breakfast Bacon Strips.

356. Make a healthier version of chicken salad using tempeh. This Mock Chicken Salad is delicious and is wonderful between two slices of whole wheat bread, in a pita pocket, rolled into a flour tortilla, or stuffed into a scooped-out tomato half.

8 ounces tempeh, any variety
¼ cup soy mayonnaise
2 teaspoons yellow mustard
1 teaspoon reduced-sodium soy sauce
½ teaspoon garlic powder
¼ teaspoon turmeric
¼ teaspoon paprika
½ cup finely chopped celery (leaves and stems)
¼ cup chopped green onion

1. Steam the tempeh over a pot of boiling water or in a vegetable steamer for about 20 minutes to make it soft enough to work with. Cool it completely, then cut or crumble the tempeh into small pieces in a medium-sized bowl.
2. Whisk together the mayonnaise, mustard, soy sauce, garlic powder, turmeric, and paprika in a small dish.
3. When the tempeh is cool, add the celery, onion, and the mayonnaise mixture, and toss everything together well. Cover and chill before serving.

357. Try sandwich fillings made with nonfat or very low fat cottage cheese as the base. The cottage cheese holds the other ingredients together. Experiment to find ingredients you like. Here are a few of my personal favorites.

358. Cottage cheese mixed with chopped walnuts, cinnamon, dates, or raisins, and a little maple syrup

359. Cottage cheese and apple butter or mashed banana

360. Cottage cheese mixed with fresh vegetables such as chopped cucumbers, bell peppers, celery, green onions, and grated carrots

361. Pita is the bread of choice when the sandwich filling is messy enough to fall out from between two slices of bread. I mentioned some pita pocket fillers earlier. Here are some more I love.

362. Baby spinach leaves tossed with grated carrots, mushrooms, garbanzo beans, red onions, sunflower seeds, and dried cherries or cranberries. Drizzle poppyseed dressing immediately before eating.

363. Scrambled egg whites with sautéed peppers and onions. I make my own using tofu in place of egg and scramble it with peppers, onions, turmeric, and a little soy sauce (see the recipe for Peppers and Tofu Scrambler on page 73).

364. Tofu egg salad (see the recipe on page 135), grated fresh vegetables such as carrots, yellow squash, cucumbers, and bell peppers.

365. Refried beans with cooked rice, chopped lettuce and tomato, and a scoop of salsa.

366. Replace luncheon meats with meatless substitutes. Natural foods stores carry a wide range of soy-based products that replace bologna and other sliced meats. You'll find some in conventional supermarkets, too. Lightlife Foods and Yves Fine Foods are two companies that make some delicious vegetarian lunch meat products. Not only are they free of trans fat, saturated fat, and cholesterol, but they're also lower in sodium than conventional luncheon meats and contain no nitrites or nitrates.

367. Instead of grilling sandwiches by slathering bread with butter or margarine, try using a panini grill or sandwich press. Nonstick grills can be sprayed with olive oil, if necessary, to prevent sticking. The device seals together the two slices of bread and the sandwich filling, and cooks the crust to a golden brown. Find panini presses in cookware specialty stores and online sources such as Williams-Sonoma and Sur La Table.

The Snack Cart

368. **Read nutrition facts labels on packaged crackers and other snack products carefully.** As this book goes to print, many companies are reformulating their snack lines to replace partially hydrogenated vegetable oils with canola oil and other trans-fat-free ingredients. For example, Kraft/Nabisco is selling trans-fat-free Triscuits, and Pepperidge Farm is making trans-fat-free Goldfish.

369. **Also make sure to scrutinize portion sizes listed on snack food labels.** Nutrition information for microwave popcorn is often listed for one-cup serving sizes. When was the last time you stopped at one cup? One or 2 grams of bad fat may not sound like much, but multiply that by two or three or more, and it begins to add up. Always make sure the serving size is reasonable, and if it's not, estimate the true serving size and multiply bad fat levels accordingly.

370. Pretzels get the "all clear." They're trans-fat-free.

371. **Have you tried crisp breads?** These crunchy flat breads (more like large crackers) originated in Sweden and are sold in most supermarkets. They're made with whole rye flour and have a slightly sour flavor. Try Wasa, Ry Krisp, Ryvita, Kavli, and Finn Crisp. I like mine smeared with raspberry preserves. Manischewitz Whole Wheat Matzos is another good product.

372. **Other good bets for an all-purpose cracker** include Nabisco Garden Herb and Roasted Garlic Triscuits, Whole Foods 365 Baked Woven Wheats, and Trader Joe's Woven Wheats Wafers.

373. Perhaps surprisingly, most brands of potato chips and tortilla chips contain no trans fat. Load them up with sour cream dip or cheese sauce, though, and you'll pile on the saturated fat.

374. Nibbles don't have to be boring. All of the following have fewer than 200 calories per serving and contain no trans fat and little or no saturated fat.

375. A frozen fruit juice bar

376. One large piece of fresh fruit

377. A half cup of whole-grain cold cereal with skim milk

378. 8 ounces of flavored soy milk

379. Half of a peanut butter and banana sandwich on whole wheat bread

380. 6 ounces of flavored low-fat or nonfat yogurt

381. A homemade bran muffin

382. 1 cup of cooked oatmeal with cinnamon, raisins, and skim milk

383. 1 cup of lentil, black bean, or split pea soup

384. 4 to 6 pieces of vegetable sushi

385. One of the best values in town is the hummus at Costco. Find it refrigerated in the deli foods section in one-pound tubs for a fraction of the price you'd pay at the supermarket. Hummus is an ultra-healthy snack food. Use it as a dip for tortilla chips and raw veggies or scoop it with toasted pita points.

386. Fruit salad drizzled with honey-yogurt sauce is a sweet and refreshing snack. Also try adding some fresh mint from the garden.

BONUS TIP: It is hard to eat while you're jogging around the block or riding your bike. Exercise helps control your appetite and keeps you healthy and in shape. Make time for it every day.

387. Flavor popcorn without adding trans fat or saturated fat: Spritz hot popcorn lightly with olive oil from a small plant mister or bottle made for that purpose (such as a product called Misto). Then sprinkle the popcorn with chili powder, cayenne pepper, garlic powder, or another favorite herb or spice mixture. Toss well.

388. Develop some strategies that will help you resist the temptation to visit the vending machines when hunger strikes at the office. Maintain a personal emergency snack stash. Trans-fat-free snacks that keep well in a desk drawer include bags of dried fruit, individual servings of canned fruit, nuts, pretzels, and soup cups or hot cereal cups. Keep a supply of disposable spoons on hand. If you are watching your weight and are concerned that having food at your desk may lead to unnecessary snacking, move your supply to a file cabinet across the room or another location that makes it a bit less convenient. Just be sure to store any loose food such as nuts or pretzels in airtight containers or plastic bags to keep bugs out.

389. Also think about keeping fresh fruit on hand. Maintaining a permanent fruit bowl with oranges, apples, pears, or bananas is not only good insurance against snack emergencies, but it also encourages you to get regular doses of nutritious, filling, low-calorie fruits that most of us would benefit from eating more often. You'll be doing a good deed if you make your fruit bowl available to coworkers as well.

390. Bring bits and pieces from home. Make it a daily habit to bring a lunch bag filled with small amounts of leftover food from home. Do that, and you can graze throughout the day on food that is more likely to be good for you. Small servings of leftover vegetables, salads, bread, cut-up vegetables, a whole tomato from the garden—all these make good between-meal snacks away from home. Bring enough so that you have snacks for mid-morning and late afternoon, the times when you are most likely to need a lift.

391. As for the vending machine, things may actually be looking up soon. Companies are beginning to stock healthier options. Canteen Vending Services, which maintains vending machines in businesses and industries throughout North America, is adding to some of its machines food, snacks, and beverages that are low in fat, sodium, and sugar, according to Kim Salahie, director of culinary development. Among the additions are hot and cold cereals, granola bars, low-fat/low-sodium popcorn, soups, salads, vegetable slices with low-fat dressing, fresh whole fruit and sliced fruit, dried fruit, nuts, yogurt, smoothies, 100 percent juice, and organic coffee.

392. Remember, you have the ultimate control over what you eat and what you avoid. Thinking through your options and planning ahead are your best defense against impulsive or less than healthy choices.

393. Keep an airtight container of ready-to-eat veggies in your refrigerator. Store them on the top shelf where you'll see them first when you open the door. If they're washed and ready, I'll choose celery sticks with peanut butter as a quick snack anytime. Broccoli and cauliflower florets, carrot sticks, and green pepper slices are light and refreshing with peach salsa or guacamole. Set them out and watch them disappear.

BONUS TIP: The fresh mango salsa at Costco is another excellent value. It's delicious used as a dip for tortilla chips or raw vegetables, over a bean burrito, on a veggie burger, or in a southwestern egg white omelet.

Appetizers and Hors d'Oeuvres

394. Bruschetta is a simple and elegant appetizer. To make it, brush baguette slices with olive oil and top with chopped fresh tomato, basil, and a sprinkling of grated low-fat cheese. Toast in the oven until melted.

395. A bruschetta variation is to spread pesto on baguette slices and top with chopped fresh tomato tossed with chopped walnuts and grated low-fat cheese. Toast in the oven until melted. The bonus: Your house will smell divine.

396. Also try adding thin strips of roasted red pepper, sun-dried tomatoes, or sliced black olives.

397. In lieu of cheese balls, serve antipasto platters. Try creating colorful arrangements of roasted peppers, marinated mushrooms, fresh sliced vegetables, an assortment of olives, basil leaves, and sun-dried tomatoes. Add salsa, hummus, black bean dip, and blended yogurt and spinach or artichoke dips, along with French bread rounds, flatbreads, whole-grain crackers, and bread sticks for scooping.

398. Fruit kebabs make a sunny and light treat. Place chunks of melon, fresh pineapple, banana, kiwi, strawberries, and grapes on wooden skewers. Dip the banana in lemon or orange juice first to delay browning.

399. Hot soup makes a comforting appetizer while friends hang out in the kitchen waiting for dinner. Try tomato basil,

Chinese hot and sour, Japanese miso, or potato leek. Serve soup in mugs with crunchy bread sticks for dipping.

400. **Baba ghanoush** (ba-ba-ga-NOOSH) is a smooth, creamy dip or spread with a mild garlicky flavor. A traditional Middle Eastern food, it is made with roasted eggplant prepared in a food processor or blender. Use it like hummus as a dip for pita points or raw vegetables, stuff it into a pita pocket, or use it as a sandwich spread.

401. **Make baba ghanoush yourself at home.** It's easy. First, slice a medium eggplant in half lengthwise. Place both halves in an oiled baking dish, insides down, and cover the dish with foil. Bake at 350 degrees for an hour, until the eggplant is soft. Let it cool, then scoop out the seeds and remove the outer peel with a paring knife. Place the remaining eggplant in a food processor or blender, add 3 tablespoons sesame tahini, 2 teaspoons minced garlic, 3 tablespoons lemon juice, and ¼ cup finely chopped parsley. Blend until smooth. Transfer the dip to a serving bowl and chill for a couple of hours before serving.

402. Who said appetizers had to be rich and fattening to taste good? **For a change of pace, serve a chilled, creamy fruit soup before dinner (or as a snack or for breakfast**—anytime!). In a blender, combine the flesh of a medium cantaloupe cut into chunks, 1 cup freshly squeezed orange juice, the juice from 1 freshly squeezed lemon or lime, 1 tablespoon honey, and 1 cup plain nonfat yogurt. Process until smooth, then pour into clear glass bowls or cups. Garnish with fresh mint leaves. Makes four servings. For a delicious adult variation, replace part of the orange juice with champagne or sparkling wine.

403. **Sometimes an appetizer or two can be all you need for a light meal.** A few pieces of bruschetta, some marinated mushrooms, or a cup of bean soup may satisfy your hunger without loading on the calories and trans fat.

404. Two cookbooks especially rich in ideas for healthy appetizers and hors d'oeuvres are *Vegetarian Times Vegetarian Entertaining* (Macmillan, 1996) and *1,000 Vegetarian Recipes,* by Carol Gelles (Macmillan, 1996).

405. Chinese boiled vegetable dumplings (also called pot stickers) make a unique and satisfying hors d'oeuvre free of bad fats. Try serving them with hot tea for a traditional and delicious before-meal dish.

406. Small wraps can be an appetizer or a light meal. Wrap warmed tomato or spinach flour tortillas around strips of barbecued tofu and steamed grated carrots, onions, zucchini, and green pepper strips.

407. Top black bean cakes with a dollop of mango or peach salsa and a teaspoon of fat-free sour cream. No time to make your own? Substitute Morningstar Farms Black Bean Burger patties, which are available in most supermarkets.

Chapter 11

Get the Trans Fat Out of
Desserts, Baked Goods, and Treats

When it comes to identifying sources of trans fat in your diet, sweet treats are the mother lode. In addition to restaurant foods, which we'll cover in the next chapter, desserts, sweets, and baked goods are where you should focus most of your attention. That's because whether you make them yourself at home, buy them from the store, or eat them when you're out, the ways these foods are traditionally prepared makes them rich sources of bad fats, both trans and saturated.

But don't worry—you don't have to give up dessert forever. For starters, there are many ingredient substitutions you can make in home recipes to radically reduce or eliminate bad fats from your favorite baked goods and desserts. Homemade is nearly always best. Make it yourself at home, and you have control over what goes into your food.

It's not hard to do. I had an "ah-ha!" moment many years ago, and I haven't needed to use bad fats in my cooking since.

As a kid, I enjoyed the popular television show *Gilligan's Island*, the '70s sitcom about a boatful of castaways marooned on a deserted tropical island. A budding baker, I was mesmerized by the coconut cream pies and banana cream pies the characters were somehow able to make despite the fact that they had no access to eggs, milk, butter, or margarine. Well, okay, they had coconut milk on the island, but still . . . It was a puzzle to me how they pulled off making those mouthwatering desserts.

Years later I learned about food chemistry in college and became aware of the specific functions of ingredients in foods—how ingredients interact with one another, the principles of leavening and browning, how ingredients can bind or moisten foods, and so on. It wasn't until I developed an interest in vegetarian diets, though, that it all clicked for me. I began working with vegans—people who eat no animal products whatsoever—and was exposed to some talented chefs and cookbook writers who could make delicious soups, breads, entrees, and desserts exclusively with plant-based ingredients. As a dietitian, the big bonus I saw was that the foods were totally free of saturated fat and cholesterol, and most were healthier in other ways, too. They were lower in added sugar and salt, and higher in fiber. Most, it turned out, were also free of trans fat.

Many of the tips I have to share with you come from the vegetarian and natural foods traditions, because they are naturally healthier for you. They seem a little odd at first, but they work. For example, just ¼ cup of tofu blended with the liquid ingredients in most recipes can replace a whole egg.

All the foods described in this chapter taste great, but it is true that recipes modified to remove bad fats often produce foods that have a somewhat different flavor, texture, or consistency than the original. You may need to experiment a bit to find which ideas work for your tastes and which don't. Keep open-minded expectations when you're trying new recipes. Your taste preferences will likely adapt to new ingredients so that you don't notice the differences anymore or even prefer the new versions.

This has certainly been true for me. For instance, I now bake cookies using vegetable oil instead of margarine, and I don't notice a difference in the finished products. There are recipes in which oil doesn't work—shortbread cookies, for example—so I don't make them anymore. But whole-grain ranger cookies and oatmeal cookies are no problem. On the other hand, I also make piecrust using vegetable oil instead of solid shortening, and I do notice the difference. Piecrust made with oil is denser and not as flaky as it would be if made with original Crisco. But I actually like the healthier version of my piecrust; I've adapted.

In this chapter, then, you'll find simple ways you can modify your favorite recipes and prepare great-tasting baked goods, desserts, and treats with minimal or zero bad fats. You will also find other strategies for minimizing your exposure to bad fats from these foods, along with commercial products you can buy if you don't have the time or inclination to make your own.

Fabulous Fruits

408. **Fruits are nature's original dessert.** Fresh figs, sweet dates, bananas, oranges, mangoes, persimmons, and pineapples are perfectly nutritious. They're 100 percent free of bad fats, and they can do a great job of satisfying a sweet tooth. Just make them available so that they come to mind when you feel like eating something sweet. Keep a large bowl of fruit on the kitchen counter, and keep washed and sliced fruits on the top shelf of the refrigerator where they're always handy. When fresh fruit threatens to spoil before you can eat it, cut it up and toss a quick fruit salad. You'll be more likely to eat it, and the fruit won't go to waste.

409. **For a taste of the tropics, eat a papaya!** Slice it in half, scoop out and discard the black seeds, squeeze the juice of a fresh lime over it, and dig in.

BONUS TIP: Ripe papayas are yellow and green and soft to the touch, like a ripe peach or pear. Some varieties of papaya can grow quite large—as big as melons. Larger papayas are often sold by the pound in countries outside the United States and in some ethnic food markets. The variety most commonly sold in the United States is typically no bigger than a large pear and sold individually.

410. Expect to get a little messy the first time you eat a mango. They have to be peeled, which can take some practice. They're slippery, and you'll have to maneuver around the pit. It is worth it, though, because the mango is one of the sweetest, most delicious of fruits. The peels of ripe mangoes are partly yellow and may have orange, red, and even black areas on them. A ripe mango "gives" slightly when pressed with thumb and forefinger.

BONUS TIP: To eat a mango, follow these steps:

1. Wash the mango.

2. Cut the mango in half lengthwise using a serrated knife. Be careful to work around the large, flat pit that lies in the center of the fruit. When you've cut the mango in half, the side with the pit will be the larger half.

3. Cut the pit out of the larger half of the mango.

4. One half at a time, hold the mango in your hand with the peel side down and the fruit inside facing upward. Using the knife, carefully score it in a crisscross pattern so that each half has been cut into cubes down to the peel but not penetrating it.

5. Set down the knife. With both hands, hold the sides of one of the mango halves and turn it inside out. The fruit cubes should push away from the peel, fanning out so that you can take bites without getting your face messy. Another option is to cut the cubes off the peel and eat them individually.

411. Apples add moisture, sweetness, and fiber to baked goods without adding bad fats. Grate apples and add them to quick breads, muffins, and pancakes. You can even use applesauce to replace part or all of the fat in baked goods. Muffins made this way are spongier in texture than they would ordinarily be, but they taste great. Try using half the butter or margarine the recipe calls for and substituting applesauce for the other half.

412. Another great apple dessert option is a baked apple topped with nonfat vanilla yogurt, cinnamon, and brown sugar.

413. Or make apple crisp, which is sweetened apples baked and topped with oatmeal crumble made from whole oats, flour, brown sugar, and oil. It has fewer calories and all the taste of apple pie or apple cobbler without the trans fat that is in a typical pie- or pastry crust.

414. Frozen bananas are another great dessert option. Freeze ripened bananas in the peel or keep peeled bananas in freezer bags. Eat them as is or blended into smoothies. Some heavy-duty blenders and juicers will process frozen bananas into a creamy, soft-serve-like treat that is out-of-this-world delicious. No other ingredients are necessary.

415. Frozen grapes are sweet and refreshing on a hot summer day. Another option is to slice fresh pineapple into one-inch-thick slabs and freeze for a fresh treat.

416. Serve fresh raspberries in a chilled champagne glass for an elegant dessert. Serve plain or top with a dollop of nonfat vanilla yogurt. And here are some other options for beautiful and healthy desserts:

417. *Ripe strawberries* dipped into powdered sugar

418. *Sweet blueberries* topped with a scoop of nonfat vanilla yogurt

419. A sliced *banana* topped with nonfat coffee yogurt

420. *Papaya, mango,* and *pineapple chunks* garnished with fresh mint leaves

421. Set out a plate of freshly sliced orange wedges at the end of a meal. Juicy, sweet oranges are just enough after a full dinner.

422. Make your own frozen juice poppers by filling ice tray molds with fruit juice and freezing until solid. Pop the mini juice bars out of the molds and store them in the freezer in airtight plastic bags for a quick sweet treat later.

Tips for Better Baking

423. To most nutritionists, Crisco shortening has always been almost synonymous with trans fat, but not anymore. A new formulation mixes fully hydrogenated cottonseed oil—a hard, waxy substance—with sunflower and soy oils to soften it into a form that resembles the appearance and function of original Crisco shortening. The new product, Crisco Zero Grams Trans Fat Per Serving All-Vegetable Shortening, contains no trans fat or cholesterol. Note, though, that it contains 3 grams of saturated fat per tablespoon, so you should still use it sparingly.

424. Use nonstick cooking spray or vegetable oil in place of margarine and butter to grease baking pans. They work just as well and are usually trans-fat-free.

425. Sweet potatoes can replace part of the egg in baked goods. In recipes that call for more than one egg, use ¼ cup mashed sweet potatoes in place of one of the eggs. It cuts the cholesterol content of muffins, cookies, and quick breads. If you experiment a bit, you may find you can use mashed sweet potato in place of all the eggs in some recipes. There are other replacements for a whole egg in baked goods, too. Note that when fruit purees replace egg, the finished product may be a bit denser than usual, but you can add an extra ½ teaspoon baking powder to lighten the product. Here are some very good egg replacements:

426. Half of a small, *ripe banana*, mashed

427. ¼ cup *applesauce*, canned pumpkin, or pureed prunes. (Depending on the recipe, these may add a bit of their distinct flavors.)

428. 1 heaping tablespoon *soy flour or bean flour* mixed with 1 tablespoon water

429. 2 tablespoons *cornstarch* beaten with 2 tablespoons water

430. 1 tablespoon finely *ground flaxseeds* whipped with ¼ cup water. (The flax is also a good source of omega-3 fatty acids.)

431. Sometimes you can omit the egg. Baked goods that are flat, such as pancakes and cookies, don't rely on eggs for lift or leavening. In these cases, eggs can often be left out of the recipes without noticeably affecting the final products. That is particularly likely to be true when a recipe calls for only one egg. If you do omit an egg, replace it with 1 to 2 tablespoons of any liquid, such as water, soy milk, or fruit juice, to maintain the proper moisture level in the food.

432. In recipes that call for whole milk, use skim or ½ percent milk instead to lower the combined level of trans fat and saturated fat. You can also substitute soy milk or rice milk cup for cup in any recipe.

BONUS TIP: Natural foods stores also sell almond milk, oat milk, and potato milk, all of which can be used cup for cup instead of cow's milk in recipes for baked goods. These milks are less popular than soy milk and rice milk, but they're good options for people with allergies or intolerances to cow's milk or soybeans.

433. Soy yogurt is a saturated-fat-free replacement for dairy yogurt. It can be used in most of the ways dairy yogurt can be used, including in recipes for cakes and quick breads. The possible exception is recipes that require the yogurt to be cooked on the stove (in puddings or sauces, for example). In that case, some separation may occur with soy yogurt. In cold recipes (fruit soups or dips, for instance), separation is not a problem.

434. You can make a version of buttermilk that contains no trans fat or saturated fat to use in recipes. Add 2 teaspoons of lemon juice or vinegar to 1 cup of soy milk or other nondairy milk replacer, and you'll have a bad-fat-free replacement.

435. You can cut the fat in most recipes by at least one-third without adversely affecting the flavor. Just add one-third less butter or margarine to the recipe. If you do, replace the fat you remove with applesauce, mashed banana, pureed prunes, or mashed pumpkin or sweet potato. The end product will be spongier or chewier than the original, but if that doesn't bother you, who cares?

436. Hodgson Mills makes a wonderful trans-fat-free whole wheat gingerbread mix. You can find it at most supermarkets. And natural foods stores carry a wide range of trans-fat-free whole-grain mixes of all kinds.

437. Boost the fiber and mineral content of quick breads and cookies you bake at home. In most cases you can replace half of the white flour with whole wheat flour. Replacing only half of the white flour shouldn't cause adverse results in the flavor of the product.

438. Don't buy large eggs. Buy only small or medium eggs, and you'll add less cholesterol to baked goods.

439. Expand the range of grains you use in baking. If you keep things interesting, you'll have an easier time staying motivated to do your own baking at home, and that can translate into less trans fat in your diet. Here are some unusual grains you can try.

440. *Kamut* (kah-MOOT) is a type of wheat with roots in ancient Egypt. In Europe it has been used for generations to make baked goods.

441. *Spelt* is another wheat used in Europe for baking. You can use it in most of the same ways that you use wheat flour, with one exception: If you are making yeast breads, spelt (as well as kamut) has to be mixed with another kind of flour for the bread to rise. Spelt is low in gluten, a protein that gives yeast bread its structure and traps the gases produced by the yeast, allowing the bread to rise. Low-gluten flour used on its own creates bread that won't hold its shape or is too dense.

442. *Teff* is one of the oldest cultivated grains. It is used in Ethiopia to make injera, a delicious large, round, flat, spongy bread that is a staple there. If you eat in an Ethiopian restaurant, you'll be served injera folded like a napkin into quarters. Rip off small pieces and use them to pinch bite-sized bits of food. Teff is also used as a whole-grain cooked cereal, and the flour can be used to make breads, muffins, and pancakes.

Pies and Puddings

443. Omit the crust if you can. Pies made the traditional way are high in trans fat and/or saturated fat thanks to the lard, solid shortening, butter, or margarine used to make the crust. You can avoid that problem by omitting the crust altogether for pies with a filling that can hold its shape without a crust, such as pumpkin or sweet potato pie. Just pour the filling into a baking dish to make a crustless pie or "pudding."

444. Use vegetable oil to make your own trans-fat-free pie-crust. To make a basic crust for an 8- or 9-inch pie, stir ⅓ cup vegetable oil with 1 cup flour and ½ teaspoon salt. Sprinkle in up to 3 tablespoons cold water, 1 tablespoon at a time, mixing with a fork until the flour is moistened and the dough forms a ball. If the dough seems dry, add another tablespoon or two of oil. Press the dough into a ball, then flatten and roll it out to the appropriate size.

445. Try this easy and delicious recipe:

Maple Pumpkin Pecan Pie

PREP TIME: 15 MINUTES
COOKING TIME: 40 MINUTES

Yield: 6 servings

One 15-ounce can (about 2 cups) pumpkin or sweet potato
8 ounces silken firm tofu
½ cup pure maple syrup
½ teaspoon ground ginger
1 teaspoon cinnamon
¼ teaspoon nutmeg
1 tablespoon flour
One 9-inch ready-made, trans-fat-free piecrust
¼ cup chopped pecans or walnuts

(continued)

1. Preheat the oven to 350 degrees. In a blender or food processor, puree the pumpkin or sweet potato, tofu, maple syrup, ginger, cinnamon, nutmeg, and flour.
2. Pour the filling into the pie shell and sprinkle nuts across the top.
3. Bake for 40 minutes, or until the filling is set. Cool and serve.

For a crustless pie you can pour the filling into an oiled 8 by 8-inch baking dish and bake as directed. It will keep its shape even without the crust.

446. Try a fruit crisp. Berry pies and one-crust pies tend to be lower in bad fats than cream pies and pies with two crusts. But fruit crisps, with no crust whatsoever, tend to be lower in bad fats than all of the above. My very favorite berry dessert—a cobbler, in this case—comes from Jennifer Raymond's cookbook, *The Peaceful Palate*. It's quick and easy to make, and it's absolutely delicious.

Berry Cobbler

5 to 6 cups fresh or frozen berries (boysenberries, blackberries, raspberries, or a mixture)
3 tablespoons whole wheat flour
½ cup plus 2 tablespoons sugar
1 cup whole wheat pastry flour
1½ teaspoons baking powder
¼ teaspoon salt
2 tablespoons vegetable oil
½ cup soy milk or rice milk

Preheat the oven to 400 degrees. Spread the berries in a 9 by 9-inch baking dish. Mix in the whole wheat flour and

½ cup sugar. In a separate bowl, mix the pastry flour and the remaining 2 tablespoons sugar with the baking powder and salt. Add the oil to the flour mixture and mix it with a fork or your fingers until the mixture resembles coarse cornmeal. Add the soy milk or rice milk and stir to combine. Spread this mixture over the berries (don't worry if they're not completely covered) and bake for about 25 minutes, or until golden brown.

447. You can substitute soy milk or rice milk cup for cup for low-fat or whole cow's milk in pudding recipes, thereby lowering your combined trans fat and saturated fat.

448. Imagine Foods Dream Pudding is a delicious, creamy nondairy dessert with no trans fat or saturated fat. It is sold in natural foods stores in packs of four single servings and comes in four flavors: chocolate, banana, butterscotch, and lemon.

Cookies and Cakes

449. For a great selection of trans-fat-free cookies and cakes, shop at a natural foods store. Packaged baked goods sold in conventional supermarkets are notorious for containing large amounts of partially hydrogenated vegetable oils. Read product labels carefully. Remember, even if the package advertises "no trans fat," check to be sure the saturated fat content is also low or zero. As companies reformulate their products to remove the trans fat, some of them might compensate by increasing the amount of saturated fat that their products contain.

450. Products can contain partially hydrogenated oils and still show zero trans fat on the nutrition facts panel. That's because regulations permit food companies to list as zero any amounts totaling less than 0.5 gram per serving. Consider how many servings you would realistically eat. If the serving size is two cookies but you'd actually eat ten, those small quantities of trans fat could add up.

451. My favorite oatmeal cookies are easy to make and contain no trans fat or saturated fat.

Soft Oatmeal Cookies

PREP TIME: 15 MINUTES

COOKING TIME: 15 MINUTES

Yield: About 3 dozen

¾ cup vegetable oil
1 cup packed brown sugar
½ cup white sugar
½ ripe banana, mashed, or 1 egg's worth of Ener-G Egg Replacer
¼ cup water
1 teaspoon pure vanilla extract
1 cup all-purpose flour
1 teaspoon salt
1 teaspoon cinnamon
½ teaspoon baking soda
½ teaspoon ground cloves
3 cups quick-cooking oats
1 cup chopped nuts (optional)
1 cup raisins (optional)

Preheat the oven to 350 degrees and mix all the ingredients except the nuts and raisins with an electric mixer. Stir in the nuts and raisins, if using. Drop the batter by the teaspoonful about 1 inch apart onto an oiled baking sheet. Bake for 15 minutes, or until the cookies are firm to the touch. Remove from the baking sheet and let cool.

452. If you love chocolate chip cookies, eliminate all the trans fat and the majority of the saturated fat by substituting vegetable oil for butter or margarine. If you substitute carob chips for the chocolate chips, you'll also eliminate the saturated fat that is contributed by the cocoa butter in the chocolate. Try this common recipe and see for yourself.

Easy Chocolate Chip Cookies

PREP TIME: 20 MINUTES

COOKING TIME: 10 MINUTES

Yield: 7½ dozen

1 tablespoon Ener-G Egg Replacer plus 4 tablespoons water or
    1 ripe banana, mashed
⅔ cup vegetable oil
¾ cup packed brown sugar
¾ cup white sugar
1 teaspoon pure vanilla extract
2¼ cups all-purpose flour
1 teaspoon baking soda
1 teaspoon salt
One 12-ounce bag of chocolate chips or carob chips
½ cup chopped walnuts (optional)

1. Preheat the oven to 375 degrees.
2. In a small dish or cup, whisk together the Egg Replacer, then set aside.
3. In a large mixing bowl, cream together the oil, brown sugar, white sugar, and vanilla. Add the Egg Replacer and beat well. Gradually add the flour, baking soda, and salt, mixing well after each addition. Fold in the chocolate chips and nuts, if desired.
4. Drop the batter by the teaspoonful onto ungreased baking

(continued)

sheets. Bake for 8 to 10 minutes, or until lightly browned. Do not overbake.

453. Find a replacement for frosting. Ready-made cake frosting is often made with solid shortening whipped with powdered sugar, so it is loaded with trans fat. When you make cupcakes and layer cakes at home, you can decorate the tops using powdered sugar instead of frosting. Store powdered sugar for this purpose in a shaker can or simply pour a little powdered sugar from the box into a mesh strainer or colander and shake over the cake tops. For yellow and white cakes use chocolate powdered sugar or plain cocoa powder for contrast.

454. *If you are in a hurry but want something sweet,* the Six-Minute Chocolate Cake recipe in the Moosewood Collective's *Moosewood Restaurant Book of Desserts* is a lifesaver. Best of all, it doesn't contain a speck of trans fat or saturated fat. It is easy and light and delicious. The magic ingredient, vinegar, reacts with the baking soda in this recipe and helps the cake rise.

Six-Minute Chocolate Cake

PREP TIME: 6 MINUTES
COOKING TIME: 30 MINUTES

Yield: 8 servings

1½ cups unbleached white flour
⅓ cup unsweetened cocoa powder
1 teaspoon baking soda
½ teaspoon salt
1 cup sugar
½ cup vegetable oil
1 cup cold water or coffee
2 teaspoons pure vanilla extract
2 tablespoons cider vinegar

1. Preheat the oven to 375 degrees.

2. Sift together the flour, cocoa, baking soda, salt, and sugar directly into a 9-inch round or 8-inch square cake pan. (Oiling the pan is recommended.)

3. Place the oil, cold water or coffee, and vanilla in a 2-cup measuring cup and mix together. Add to the baking pan and mix with a fork or a small whisk.

4. When the batter is smooth, add the vinegar and stir quickly. There will be pale swirls in the batter as the baking soda and vinegar react. Stir just until the vinegar is evenly distributed throughout the batter.

5. Bake for 25 to 30 minutes, then set aside to cool.

The original recipe calls for an optional chocolate glaze made with chocolate chips, hot water, and vanilla. You can omit this and instead dust the cake with powdered sugar when it is cool.

455. Banana bread is delicious and healthy. A recipe that is near and dear to my heart is the banana bread from *The New Laurel's Kitchen,* by Laurel Robertson, Carol Flinders, and Brian Ruppenthal (Ten Speed Press, 1986). This can be considered a cake because it is so delectable and can be baked in a loaf, an 8-inch square pan, or a cupcake tin with 12 cups. This recipe is another example of a fabulous dessert made with no milk, eggs, or butter. It is trans-fat- and saturated-fat-free.

Banana Bread

Yield: 1 loaf

2 very ripe bananas, mashed (makes 1 cup)
Juice of 1 lemon
⅓ cup oil
½ cup brown sugar
1½ cups whole wheat flour
½ teaspoon salt
½ teaspoon baking powder
½ teaspoon baking soda
½ cup wheat germ
1 cup chopped dates (optional)
1 cup toasted nuts (optional)

1. Preheat the oven to 375 degrees.
2. Mix the mashed bananas with lemon juice until smooth.
3. Cream the oil and sugar together. Add the banana mix and stir well.
4. Sift together the flour, salt, baking powder, and baking soda. Mix in the wheat germ. Add to the banana mix, then stir in the dates and nuts if desired.
5. The dough will be very stiff. Turn it into a greased 4 by 8-inch loaf pan and bake for about 45 minutes. To test for doneness, insert a knife in the loaf. The bread is done when it comes out clean.

456. **If you've never tried tofu cheesecake, you're in for a surprise—and a treat.** Making the cake with tofu lets you enjoy all the richness without the bad fats. Check out the easy recipes for Chocolate Cheesecake, Maple Tofu Cheesecake, and others (plus photos) in *Tofu Cookery,* revised edition, by Louise Hagler (Book Publishing Company, 1991). In all these recipes the cream cheese or ricotta cheese typically used to make traditional cheesecakes is replaced with a blend of tofu, vegetable oil, lemon juice, and a pinch of salt. Honey and vanilla are used to sweeten the filling. The tofu filling isn't low in calories, but it's free of trans fat and very low in saturated fat.

Toppings and Frozen Treats

457. Whipped cream is positively crammed with bad fats. My favorite topping for fresh berries or fruit salad is a big dollop of nonfat vanilla or lemon yogurt.

458. Make a sweet dessert topping that is low in trans fat using tofu and nut milk. This recipe is easy to make, and the topping is suitable for pies, berries, cream puffs, or as a frosting. Grind 4 tablespoons cashews in a coffee grinder or food processor. Transfer the finely ground nuts to a small dish and whisk together with ½ cup water. Pour half of the cashew milk into a blender. Add 1 pound silken firm tofu, ¼ cup pure maple syrup, 1½ teaspoons pure vanilla extract, and a pinch of salt. Process until smooth, adding the remaining cashew milk as needed to achieve the desired consistency. Makes about 2 cups of topping.

459. Remember that ice cream has bad fats, too. When it comes to this sweet treat, it seems the bowl is never big enough. But when ice cream becomes a daily indulgence, the saturated fat load can push your intake of trans fat plus saturated fat to unhealthy levels. What is an ice cream lover to do? You have options.

460. Choose ice cream brands with the least amount of saturated fat per serving. Many brands hover around 2 grams of saturated fat or less per half-cup serving. Examples include Healthy Choice vanilla ice cream and Breyers 98% Fat-Free vanilla. Each has 1 gram of saturated fat per serving.

461. **Experiment with alternatives to ice cream that contain little or no saturated fat.** Good examples include sorbet, sherbet, frozen yogurt, and Italian ice. Read and compare nutrition labels. Shop around for brands you especially like. Green's nonfat frozen yogurt, for example, has a creamy texture similar to ice cream but with zero saturated fat and only 110 calories per half cup. Rice- and soy-based frozen desserts sold at natural foods stores are another good-tasting option, although they can be pricey.

462. **Watch the portion size.** A 1-cup scoop of ice cream can look deceptively small in a big cereal bowl. Be aware of how much you are eating; it's easy to eat more than you think you are.

463. **Watch what you put on top.** Hot fudge, caramel sauce, or candy bits can add substantially more saturated fat and possibly trans fat, too. If you need a topping, use fruit or sprinkles instead of fudge and other rich sauces.

464. **Avoid premium brands.** They deliver the most calories and fat. Compare the nutrition labels and see for yourself.

465. **Go out for an occasional cone** rather than bringing home a half-gallon. You'll eat less that way.

466. **Use a custard cup or small mug rather than a cereal bowl.** You'll eat less and could cut the calories and saturated fat in half.

467. **If you love ice cream, make it a weekly tradition instead of a nightly event.** If you do nothing more than switch to once a week—perhaps on a particuar night—you'll radically reduce your saturated fat and calorie intake.

468. Be aware that frozen yogurt advertised as being "96 percent fat-free" is high in saturated fat. It is 4 percent milk fat by weight, just like whole milk. Of course, whole milk is mostly water (which accounts for most of its weight). Both whole milk and low-fat frozen yogurt actually get 50 percent of their calories from fat, most of it saturated. The bottom line is that if you want frozen yogurt, make sure it's fat-free or have the sorbet instead.

Managing Sweet Temptations

469. Holidays and special occasions create a particular challenge for anyone trying to limit exposure to foods—especially sweets and treats—laden with trans fat and saturated fat. Dealing with these occasions effectively is important because lapses can be demoralizing and can cause you to lose your motivation to stick with healthy eating habits. Try getting through the tough times by eating dessert first. The rationale is that if you know you're going to have cookies or a slice of pie after a meal—regardless of how full you may be—you may save yourself even more fat in the end if the dessert dulls your appetite for other rich foods. For the meal itself, you may eat smaller portions, less food, or no other food at all. Granted, this wouldn't be a nutrition-conscious approach for the long term, but for a few days over the holidays or while you're on vacation, it won't hurt and it may help.

470. Try eating samples instead of servings. When presented with a big spread, fill your plate with a few tablespoons each of whatever foods look good, rather than heaping your plate with big helpings you'll feel compelled to finish. Once you have tasted everything, take seconds only on your favorites and only if you still have room.

471. Fill the house with fruit. Keep a big bowl of colorful fruits in full view on the kitchen counter. Toss a fresh fruit salad with a light dressing made from nonfat yogurt and a little honey and orange juice. If you feel like snacking on something sweet, grab some fruit instead of cookies and cakes. Besides, you should be aiming for at least two servings of fruit a day.

472. Take an evening walk. Talk over the day with a companion, get some fresh air, and walk off some dinner and excess treats. It is a nice way to unwind, and you'll feel better getting regular exercise, especially during the holidays and vacation times when many people overeat and are less active than usual.

473. Plan family time outdoors when everyone is in town together. Make a few trips to the playground; go bike riding, hiking, or Rollerblading; play tennis; or go for a walk in the woods, on a nature trail, or through the botanical gardens. Organize activities outside and away from the TV, video games, computer, and trays of treats. Shoo the kids outdoors and get out there with them.

474. Get a project done. Give yourself a big holiday bonus by stealing some time to plant a tree in the yard, finish up some work in the garden, clear space for your car in the garage, or clean out and organize the attic now that holiday decorations are temporarily out of the way. Be active and busy rather than sitting around and eating.

475. Take time to reflect and plan. Find a quiet corner at some point during the next holiday or vacation and think about where you stand in terms of your personal wellness goals.

Chapter 12

Get the Trans Fat Out
When You Eat Out

How often do you eat out each week? According to the Center for Science in the Public Interest, which issued a report in 2003 on links between obesity and restaurant food, most of us today spend about 46 percent of our food dollars on eating out, as compared to 26 percent in 1970. That's a lot of food money spent away from home.

It follows, then, that what we eat away from home likely has a substantial effect on our health. And, unfortunately, restaurant food tends to be much higher in saturated fat, trans fat, and sodium than food made and eaten at home. It is also lower in dietary fiber and key vitamins and minerals.

So there are many reasons to choose wisely when out. But the catch is that restaurants aren't required to list the trans fat contents of their foods. In fact, they don't have to list any nutrition information at all. Policymakers and consumer advocates are pushing for change. One bill introduced in Congress, Menu Education and Labeling (MEAL), would require all restaurant chains with twenty or more stores to list on printed menus the amounts of calories, saturated fat, trans fat, carbohydrates, and sodium in their foods. Fast-food menu boards would have to post calories. The law would affect standard selections at such restaurants as Denny's, McDonald's, Taco Bell, and Kentucky Fried Chicken.

Surveys have found that two-thirds of Americans support such a move. In fact, a campaign initiated by the New York City Health Department in 2005 goes a step further and aims specifically at getting trans fat out of restaurants in New York City. Another campaign, TransFree America, launched in 2004 by the Center for Science in the Public Interest, encourages food manufacturers to find new formulas for their products that replace trans fat with natural vegetable oils. Companies such as McDonald's and Burger King have already done this in Denmark where partially hydrogenated oils have been banned from the food supply since 2003.

Not surprisingly, the restaurant industry opposes nutrition labeling on menus. Their rationale is that it is not practical, since people often customize their orders and posted nutrition information may not apply. Plus, small independent restaurants wouldn't be able to be included because their menus change frequently, the industry says.

Some restaurants do provide nutrition information in print materials and on company Web sites. That information is of little value to most of us, though, because it is not at our fingertips when we're making decisions about what to order. Most people don't even know they can ask for such information.

What to do? This chapter will provide you with tips for making healthy, trans-fat-free choices when you go out to eat. You will also find strategies for dealing with other times you may eat out, including meals at work and school, and when you travel.

Getting What You Want

476. Ask questions when you eat out. Unless a nutrient claim is made, such as low fat or no trans fat, restaurants almost never list nutrition information for foods on their menus because they're not required to do so. In most cases the only way you'll know is by asking whether partially hydrogenated oil or other sources of bad fat have been used to prepare a dish. Ask your server. If your server can't answer your question, ask him or her to check with management or the kitchen staff.

477. Family-style chains and fast-food restaurants pre-prepare much of their food and offer less flexibility than restaurants where food is made to order. Eat at mom-and-pop or higher quality restaurants instead, and you'll be able to get veggies cooked without butter or margarine and fruit salad in place of trans-fatty fries.

478. A few restaurant chains have already taken substantial action to remove the trans fat from their foods. In November 2005 the Center for Science in the Public Interest reported the following:

479. *Au Bon Pain,* a café chain based in Boston, has removed trans fat from all cookies, bagels, and muffins and is using trans-fat-free margarine.

480. *Jason's Deli,* a sandwich and salad chain, has eliminated partially hydrogenated oils in all of its products.

481. *California Pizza Kitchen* has removed trans fat from its deep-fried menu items.

482. *Ruby Tuesday* restaurants have begun deep-frying their fried foods in heart-healthy canola oil, though their suppliers still panfry some menu items in partially hydrogenated oil.

483. *Starbucks, Friendly* ice cream restaurants, and *Popeyes* told CSPI they had *no plans to remove trans fat* from their foods.

484. Ask for what you need. When I interviewed fitness guru Jack LaLanne a few years ago, he shared with me his strategy for eating out. According to LaLanne, most people who eat out go into restaurants not knowing what they want or what is healthy and what is not. Not him. "I bring the chef over and say, 'I want the best. Here's what I want. I want a salad; very little lettuce. I want bell peppers, carrots, avocados. I want at least ten raw vegetables.' And I make them chop them up real fine," he told me. He takes his salads with oil and vinegar, and orders a salad so big he doesn't always finish it.

485. Look at menus with a creative eye. Side dishes listed with entrees can often be combined to make a delicious, healthy veggie plate meal. Just ask. Look for vegetable sides sautéed in olive oil, steamed rice, and fresh fruits.

486. Substitute when necessary. Tell your server you'd like to swap the chips or fries for a small green salad or fruit even if it costs a little more. It's worth it.

Menu Savvy

487. Order a big salad. Skip the cheese and meat, and take the dressing on the side so that you can control how much goes on the salad. Go heavy on fresh vegetables, beans, and fruit. Green salads are filling and can save hundreds of calories over sandwiches and entrees laden with bad fats.

488. Split the entree with a companion. Most restaurant portions are more than one serving. Order a cup of soup and a salad to go along with it, and you'll both be satisfied. If you want dessert, split that, too. That way, even if the food is rich in bad fats, you'll eat less of them.

489. Just because they served it to you doesn't mean you have to eat it. Take half home in a to-go box, and you'll have a heat-and-serve meal for later or to take to work.

490. Eat at natural foods cafés. Small eateries associated with natural foods stores use ingredients that meet the natural foods industry's standards. That means no ingredients made with partially hydrogenated oils.

491. Beware of fried appetizers. A batter-dipped and fried whole onion plus dipping sauce, typical of those served at many steak houses, contains a whopping 18 grams of trans fat, according to the June 1999 issue of Nutrition Action Healthletter published by the Center for Science in the Public Interest. The group also reported that an order of cheese fries served with ranch dressing contains 11 grams of trans fat plus a heart-stopping 81 grams of saturated fat.

492. Don't discount smaller amounts of trans fat in meat and dairy products. The large portion sizes served in most restaurants mean that the amount of naturally occurring trans fats in animal products can add up to substantial amounts.

493. Forgo the pastries. Cinnamon rolls, Danish pastries, tarts, scones, doughnuts, and other baked treats are slathered with margarine and are typically oozing with trans fat.

494. Limit the free breads. Greasy biscuits, corn bread, and many bread sticks are high-calorie fillers with little nutritional value and too much bad fat.

495. Aim for foods that are low in total fat, and you'll likely lessen your intake of trans fat. Salads (hold the cheese and meat) with oil-based dressings are a good bet, as are broiled seafood (hold the butter), a veggie sandwich with mustard (hold the cream cheese or mayo), and Chinese stir-fried vegetables with steamed rice.

496. **Also remember to choose kids' entrees carefully.** Avoid fried meats, chicken nuggets, hotdogs, burgers, and cheese-and-meat-laden pizzas. The best kid-friendly options are pasta with tomato sauce and entrees made with little or no meat and cheese such as bean burritos, vegetable pizza light on the cheese, and vegetable stir-fry with steamed rice. Grilled chicken or fish is better than other meats.

International Insights

497. **Entrees served at ethnic restaurants can be a good choice.** Many are based on grains and vegetables. Here are some of the best choices.

498. *Chinese:* Vegetable soup, hot and sour soup, pot stickers (steamed vegetable dumplings), Buddha's Delight (mixed vegetables with panfried bean curd), broccoli with garlic sauce, and vegetable lo mein are all safe. Ask for steamed rice and eat it liberally with your entree. Plan to take half of your meal home.

499. *Indian:* The best choices are dal (lentil soup) without ghee (butter), vegetable curries with steamed rice, and breads listed as "roti" or "naan," which are usually baked or roasted.

500. *Mexican:* Beans rule. Go for bean burritos, tacos, tostadas, and enchiladas. Add spinach or roasted vegetables if they have them. Guacamole is rich in monounsaturated fats, which are fine. Limit the artery-clogging sour cream and cheese, but you can use the salsa with abandon.

501. *Italian:* Good foods include lentil soup, minestrone soup, bruschetta, angel-hair pasta with pesto sauce, pasta primavera, and any pasta tossed with olive oil or marinara in lieu of cream sauce. Just say no to the gobs of mozzarella cheese melted on top of some pasta dishes. A sprinkling of grated Parmesan cheese is fine, though. Other good choices are pasta e fagioli (pasta with beans), green salads with vinaigrette dressing, and Italian bread dipped in olive oil. For dessert, try fresh berries or a scoop of sorbet.

502. When possible, familiarize yourself with the menu before you eat at an ethnic restaurant if it serves foods you are not used to eating. That gives you time to plan, and it may prevent impulsive choices. At the restaurant, ask questions about how unfamiliar foods are prepared before you order.

503. Eating out at ethnic restaurants has the added benefit of teaching tolerance and appreciation for other cultures. People of all ages, especially kids, can learn about geography, world history, and the art, music, and folklore of other cultures by exploring their foods. Greater familiarity can lessen fear and misunderstandings about people outside as well as within our own borders.

504. If you are new to ethnic cuisine, start with foods you know you like. If you like baked beans or pinto beans, try Indian dal, Cuban black beans and rice, or hummus. Do you like pasta? If so, then you might like Middle Eastern couscous or pasta tossed with cooked greens, garlic, olive oil, and chopped walnuts or sun-dried tomatoes.

505. In restaurants, as in the supermarket, take a chance on something new. You won't like everything you try, but you'll find some new and healthy favorites.

On the Run and on the Road

506. Eating well while you're away is important, especially if you travel often. The food you eat not only affects how you feel that day, but it also has a cumulative effect on health.

507. When you leave on a family road trip, take as much food from home as you can. You will not only save money, but you'll be better able to limit your family's exposure to bad fats. Here are some ideas on what to take in the car.

> **508.** *Sandwiches.* Use whole-grain bread. (See Chapter 10 for more tips on healthy sandwiches.) PB&Js can be pre-assembled, but store other sandwich fillings separate from the bread until it's time to eat. Tortillas and pita pockets filled with hummus may turn mushy if they're not eaten soon after you put them together.

> **509.** *Fresh fruits.* No surprise here. Take along whole apples, pears, and bananas. They'll stay fresh longer if you keep them out of the sun. Melon cubes and washed berries will keep for a couple of days if you store them in airtight containers and keep them in a cooler.

> **510.** *Portable foods that keep a long time.* Take along individually wrapped snacks such as small bags of peanuts and sunflower seeds, pretzels, dried fruit, and granola bars. I buy Nature Valley Chewy Trail Mix Fruit & Nut Bars, a better choice than most because they're made with whole oats and contain no trans fat. They also taste good.

511. On family trips that require several days at a motel, consider finding one with kitchenettes in the rooms. Stop at the local supermarket and buy what you need to make a big tossed salad and a simple dinner. You can pick up breakfast supplies there, too, and restock your stash of snacks, especially fruit.

512. **If you stop to eat when you're on the road, choose the restaurant wisely.** Remember that foods at family chain restaurants are typically loaded with trans fats, saturated fats, and sodium that may not be readily apparent by menu descriptions and pictures. In lieu of sandwiches and entrees, look for healthy side dishes you can put together for a meal, such as whole wheat toast, a green salad, a baked potato, the steamed vegetable of the day, or a bowl of broth-based soup.

513. **When you eat meals while on the road, share with your family or others.** Split entrees and order separate side salads. What's the worst that can happen? If you're still hungry, you can order more or have a piece of fruit later.

514. **Eat fewer meals when you're traveling.** Many people find that when they're on vacation, all they really need is breakfast and dinner. Especially when you're in the car and not moving around much, you don't need as much food to get you through the day. Skip lunch and save calories, bad fats, and money.

515. **If you have to stop at fast-food restaurants, raise the fiber quotient and minimize the grease factor by choosing wisely.** A Wendy's baked potato and garden salad with vinaigrette dressing on the side or a Taco Bell bean burrito or two are good choices. Generally, avoid the sandwiches and fries and order fresh fruits and vegetables if you can get them, minus any fatty toppings and with dressings on the side.

516. **Plan for layovers and delays when you travel by plane.** One traveler's defense is to eat just before leaving home. It'll hold you for a while and reduce the amount you'll need to buy at airport food courts. Eat something substantial and healthy. If you have a morning flight, give yourself enough time for a bowl of oatmeal or peanut butter on whole wheat toast and a glass of juice. Set the alarm clock a half hour earlier. You can sleep on the plane.

517. Bring a snack with you to the airport. Take dried fruit and sturdy fresh fruits such as apples and pears that won't turn to mush in your carry-on bag. Bring nuts, trail mix, or a PB&J on whole-grain bread. You can snack when you're hungry, and if there's a layover, you'll get through it without having to eat at the airport.

518. Ask yourself if you really need to eat. Can you wait until you arrive at your destination?

519. If you must eat at the airport, choose the best of the worst. A bagel is better than a doughnut, and nonfat frozen yogurt is better than a candy bar. Of course, if you can look past the pizza and pastries, you can usually spot some truly good choices—apples and bananas, fresh fruit cups, nuts— if you keep an eye out for them.

520. Larger airports are likely to have a greater number of healthy food choices. One of my all-time favorites is the black beans and rice dish at La Carreta Cuban Cuisine at the Miami International Airport. And here are some other good choices.

521. The BK Veggie Burger at Burger King. Some restaurants carry it; some don't.

522. A Wendy's baked potato and side salad. Keep the dressing on the side and use a fraction of what comes in the packet.

523. Bean burritos anywhere you can find them. Taco Bell bean burritos are fine. At the Dallas–Fort Worth airport, head to Los Amigos. My favorite is Maui Taco at the Raleigh-Durham Airport. They also have a store in the Newark International Airport. Their veggie burritos and soft tacos are also filling, delicious, and good for you. As airport food goes, they're inexpensive, too.

Cubicle Cuisine

524. Bring food from home to eat at the office. Most often it will be cheaper and better for you than trying to procure food at nearby restaurants. Bring your lunch in a small cooler or an insulated lunch bag. Pack food the night before in reusable plastic or glass single-serving containers. Good choices include the following:

525. Leftover salads, casseroles, soups, baked potatoes, and cooked vegetables

526. Seasonal fresh fruit. Even if you take nothing else, pack two to three pieces of fruit every day.

527. Fresh veggies from the garden such as cherry tomatoes, green pepper slices, and radishes. No garden? Bring prewashed baby carrots, cucumber slices, and other fresh vegetables from the store.

528. Hummus and pita bread wedges for dipping

529. Peanut butter or almond butter on whole-grain crackers

530. Soup or hot cereal cups. Just add hot water and stir.

531. Whole-grain muffins and quick breads (homemade using vegetable oil), and bagels with fruit in them. These are usually sweet enough that they don't need added cream cheese.

532. Make it easier to pack your own lunch by having some basic lunch box supplies on hand, including an insulated lunch bag or box. The biggest mistake is getting something too small. Find one with ample space to hold a squat thermos bottle or an ice pack or two in addition to food. Here are other supplies that are handy to have as well.

533. *Frozen gel packs.* Keep two or three small ones on hand, about the size of a 4-by-6 index card, and put them in lunches to keep things cool and fresh.

534. *Reusable containers.* If food is to be heated in a microwave oven, consider using glass. Otherwise, lightweight, inexpensive plastic containers—some round and some square—are what you need. Each should be able to hold a sandwich or a cup or two of food.

535. *A short thermos bottle.* It should fit into most lunch bags. These are the best choice for carrying soup, chili, and hot leftovers.

536. If you are packing a school lunch for your child, involve your kids in planning what to pack. But don't just ask them what they want in their school lunch. Give them choices and take them grocery shopping. Let them pack their own lunch the night before if they are old enough to do it.

537. Vary the foods in your kids' school lunches. Include a variety of flavors, colors, textures, and temperatures. It makes for a much more appealing meal. Think about it. Which would you rather eat? A PB&J on white bread with a bag of chips, a carton of milk, and a cookie, or a thermos-ful of chili, a handful of whole-grain crackers, a bag of green pepper slices, and orange wedges?

538. Be sure to pack in nutrition when sending your kids off for the day. The best way to do that is by including fresh fruits and vegetables and limiting foods high in bad fats.

539. Be careful at snack stands and food carts; they offer limited choices. Whole-grain breads are harder to find, and ready-made sandwiches are likely to contain fillings with mayo that are high in saturated fat. Commercial muffins and snack foods are often loaded with trans fat. Here are your best bets if they're available.

540. *Fresh fruit.* Buy more than one piece!

541. *Green salads,* fruit salad, and small bags of toasted seeds or nuts.

542. For good measure, *steer clear of soft drinks and sweetened fruit beverages* such as Snapple and Fruitopia. Buy bottled water instead or fill a glass from the drinking fountain in your office.

543. Be very careful when buying from a vending machine. Some workplaces have vending machines that dispense fresh fruit and bottled water, so they're not always a total loss. But usually they offer very little of value and lots that can do you harm. The best of the worst include fig newtons, gingersnaps, seeds and nuts, and granola bars. If you must eat from the machines, then supplement it with something from home, too—at the least fresh fruit.

544. Why not keep a bowl of fresh fruit in your office so that you have something good to eat in a pinch? Look at it this way: You can eat apples, pears, and grapes one-handed while answering e-mail. And if you're the boss, set out a big communal office fruit bowl. You'll be doing your employees a big service.

Chapter 13

Get the Trans Fat Out
of Your Life

In the years I've spent counseling individuals on diet changes, my observation has been that slow and steady is the most comfortable way for most people to change their lifestyles. Changes made gradually seem to be more likely to stick. Spreading changes out over time allows your diet to evolve as you master new ways of eating and cooking. You can get educated about how to shop and plan meals, and gain confidence in your ability to make wise choices when you eat out.

Making lifestyle changes gradually is generally less disruptive to your daily routine, too, since it gives you more time to adapt to changes each step of the way. But there are pitfalls as well. Drag out the changes, and you may get stuck in a rut along the way when you're only halfway to healthy eating habits. Habitual procrastinators are especially vulnerable. Don't let this happen to you. Have a plan to keep moving. Your plan may even include dates that you've set to reach small goals on your path to the big goal of better eating.

When you overhaul your diet—a necessity for most of us if we want to get the trans fat out—you need to gain skills and knowledge in the following:

- Nutrition and health
- Grocery shopping and stocking your home with healthy staples
- Meal planning and fixing new recipes
- More scratch cooking and planning ahead
- Eating out and while traveling
- Establishing new traditions for holidays and special occasions

I've shared lots of ways to accomplish these goals in this book. As you get started, approach the changes in a manner that makes sense for you. As you do, keep these tips in mind as well.

◆ *Break it up.* A large task can seem overwhelming when you think about it in its entirety, so don't try to make all your changes at once. Instead, write down a series of small steps that lead to the bigger goal of better eating habits. Examples might be ridding your pantry of foods containing trans fat, starting to eat two pieces of fresh fruit each day, cooking dinner from scratch three days a week, or trying out a natural foods store or natural foods items in your local grocery. Check these off as you complete each step. The sense of accomplishment will keep you motivated.

◆ *Make a list of easy favorite standbys.* You probably already eat a number of healthy foods, and you can often modify others to be better for you. Double up or even triple up on green salads and cooked veggies. Keep the fruit bowl full. Leave the beef out of the chili and spaghetti sauce. Dip crusty breads into olive oil and balsamic vinegar instead of margarine. Skip the cheese sauce on the broccoli and make beans and rice a once-a-week tradition.

◆ *Be easy on yourself.* Lifestyle changes can be difficult, and life introduces hurdles along the way including holidays, illnesses, and other distractions. You don't want to delude yourself into thinking you're making progress when you're not, but there's also no need to be too harsh on yourself if you have a setback now and then.

◆ *Be positive.* Some people see the joy in a challenge, and others just see the challenge. When you embark on a diet change, think about the many appealing foods you have to choose from rather than what you're leaving behind. It's all about attitude. Don't waste time thinking about what you used to eat. Move on and look ahead.

You may want to consider keeping a food diary to chart your progress. You can keep one for as little or as much time as you like. Try keeping a log of everything you eat each day for a week and file it away. A few months from now, do it again. And again in another three months. It can be interesting and encouraging to compare the "before" and "after" over time. It may also help you recognize a rut when you're in one.

The tips that follow will give you more ideas about how you can pull off the lifestyle change for keeps.

Getting Started

545. **Surround yourself with support.** If you live and work with others who have similar goals, it'll help you stay on track. It also helps if you know someone who models good eating habits and can help you troubleshoot challenges.

546. **Understand that lapses are normal.** If you fall back into your old eating pattern for a day or two, just pick up where you left off as soon as you can. Don't beat yourself up about it too much; just move forward.

547. **Remember the words of the late Vermont homesteader Helen Nearing.** In her book *Simple Food for the Good Life: An*

Alternative Cookbook (reissued by Chelsea Green Publishing Company, 1999), she advised us all to **eat simply.** She recommended "hearty, harmless food, simple and sustaining: simple foods for simple-living people, not complicated food for complex sophisticates." According to Helen, "If a recipe cannot be written on the face of a 3-by-5 card, off with its head." Here are some other words of wisdom from Helen.

548. Eat as well as you want to live. Helen's motto was: "Live hard, not soft; eat hard not soft; seek fiber in foods and in life."

549. Don't stress over meals. Helen geared her book toward "simple-living people who have other things paramount on their minds rather than culinary concerns" and "who eat to nourish their bodies and leave self-indulgent delicacies to the gourmets."

550. Enjoy food, but guard against excess. She wrote: "Cookbooks are usually designed for people who are overfed and oversupplied with food and who are looking for tasty additions to stimulate their worn-out appetites." She counseled simplicity, in part, to ward off cravings for unhealthy foods. "If you eat twice as much popcorn when it is heavily buttered and salted, why butter and salt it? Eat a moderate amount of plain popcorn and then stop."

551. Be creative in preparing meals. Helen experimented with whatever ingredients were on hand. She thought that keeping a modest amount of food in the house was preferable to an overflowing pantry. Having less "fosters more ingenuity," she said.

552. Eat foods as close to their natural state as possible. It is easier, better for your health, and you'll use fewer dishes, pans, and utensils.

553. You may eat more healthy veggies if you join a CSA farm. I mentioned CSA briefly at the beginning of this book, but it's worth a reminder. CSA stands for "community-supported agriculture." The concept came to the United States in the 1980s from Japan, where the term used is *teikei*. *Teikei* translates into "partnership" or "cooperation," but in the context of the CSA movement it means "food with the farmer's face on it." The idea is simple: Residents of a community pay a local farmer a predetermined amount of money up front. In return, they get a portion of the harvest throughout the growing season. To find one near you, consult your state or local farm stewardship association or state cooperative extension office.

554. You can also try the Alternative Farming Systems Information Center of the U.S. Department of Agriculture at www.nal.usda.gov/afsic/csa/ for more information on CSAs.

555. Or look up the Sustainable Agriculture Research and Education program at www.sare.org/csa/.

556. For a comprehensive list of national, regional, and state organizations and Web sites go to www.nal.usda.gov/afsic/csa/csaorgs.htm.

Family Matters

557. Take a more relaxed and social approach to eating. In an October 2004 essay in the *New York Times Magazine*, food writer Michael Pollan described Americans as having a "national eating disorder." He argued that although Americans are more anxious and food-obsessed than people in other nations, we're less healthy than many of our neighbors around the world who spend less time worrying about what they eat. "A well-developed culture of eating, such as you find in France or Italy," he said, "mediates the eater's relationship to food, moderating consumption even as it prolongs and deepens the pleasure of eating." To help make meals a social affair again at home, try the following:

558. Spend more time fixing meals. Given the frantic pace of most households, a practical approach may be to aim for taking extra time to fix a meal from scratch at least two or three times a week. Keep it simple by choosing meals that require few ingredients and little dependence on recipes. Toss a salad and cook some fresh vegetables. Other days of the week, eat leftovers and foods prepared ahead of time—a pot of chili cooked during the weekend or a vegetable lasagna made with a minimal amount of low-fat cheese.

559. Plan ahead. Prepare meals ahead of time if your schedule leaves little time once you get home at night. Fix a salad the night before (but don't add the croutons until you're ready to serve). Cook a pot of chili or prepare a casserole on Sunday night and reheat or cook it the next day.

560. Pay attention to presentation. Serve foods in bowls and on platters, not in their cooking pots. Add a garnish here and there. Keep yourself and your family interested in meals.

561. Recruit help. Everyone can pitch in. Kids can shuck corn and set the table. They can clear the table and do the dishes, too.

562. Ritualize dinner. Set the table, include everyone, and designate a regular time for meals.

563. Prepare the setting. Make mealtime as pleasant as possible by turning off the TV, adding some soft music, and setting out a candle or fresh flowers.

564. Protect mealtime. If evening is the best time for your family meal, make it a priority and don't let other activities interfere. I was struck last summer when, in talking with some new neighbors, I learned they had decided against registering their kids for swimming lessons because the lessons would have interfered with dinnertime.

565. Don't forget to include your children in your efforts to eat more healthily. Many children don't eat enough fruits or vegetables, and one of the most common "vegetables" chosen by kids is French fries. Since eating habits become entrenched at an early age, start your children off right. It's never too early to begin. Here is what you can do.

566. Let them choose. Whenever feasible, empower kids to choose from among a few wholesome meal or snack options. It increases the likelihood of their acceptance and meets their growing need to exercise independence.

567. Show variety. Keep a range of foods on hand that vary in color, texture, and flavor. Don't give up on any particular food. Kids are fickle: Today's reject may be tomorrow's favorite.

568. Get kids involved in preparing meals. Kids who have a hand in shopping for food and planning, preparing, and cleaning up after meals are more likely to eat the food that's served. Even toddlers can place ingredients in a pan or help shred lettuce or shuck corn.

569. Be positive. A positive attitude about food is contagious. Kids will take your cue and react toward foods accordingly.

570. Be a role model. Let kids see you enjoying the foods you'd like them to eat. And if you don't want them craving French fries, don't let them see you downing them yourself.

571. Offer acceptable substitutes for hotdogs and French fries. Instead of fries, for instance, serve oven-baked potato chunks or wedges, and instead of candy, encourage kids to snack on fresh fruit. Other healthy kid favorites include peanut butter and jelly sandwiches; mashed potatoes; raw vegetable sticks with low-fat dip; whole-grain muffins, pancakes, and waffles; flavored nonfat yogurt or soy yogurt; bean burritos; noodles with tomato sauce; and milk shakes made with frozen bananas or berries mixed with skim milk or fortified soy or rice milk.

Resources on the Web

572. Consumer's Union at **www.consumersunion.org**. This site gives unbiased advice about health and nutrition supported by sales of *Consumer Reports* magazine, related services, and noncorporate grants, contributions, and fees.

573. Harvard Nutrition Source at **www.hsph.harvard.edu/ nutritionsource/**. The site is maintained by the Department of Nutrition at the Harvard School of Public Health.

574. Nutrition Action Healthletter at **www.cspinet.org/nah**. Published by the Center for Science in the Public Interest, the site offers free online access to back issues or subscriptions to their newsletter.

575. Environmental Working Group at **www.ewg.org**. This offers reliable information on food and water safety and policy.

576. Environmental Nutrition Newsletter at **www.environ mentalnutrition.com**. Here you'll find reports on food and nutrition science and policy news from a public interest perspective. You can access current and back issues free for thirty days before opening a paid subscription.

577. The U.S. Department of Agriculture's Food and Nutrition Information Center at **www.nal.usda.gov/fnic/general/ general.html**. It provides links to other Web sites and subsites, resource lists, and A-to-Z topic information and searchable databases, including one that gives the nutrient composition of foods.

578. The National Institutes of Health at **http://health.nih. gov/**. The site has links to health databases, hotlines, and information on specific nutrition and wellness topics. You can also go directly to the National Library of Medicine at **www.nlm. nih.gov/portals/public.html** and get instructions for using the online collection.

579. Healthfinder at **www.healthfinder.gov/**. This is a federal government Web site for consumers that links to more than fifteen hundred government and nonprofit sources of health and human services information on the Web. It includes links to Spanish-language resources and offers a quick tour for anyone new to the site.

580. American Heart Association at **www.americanheart. org/**. It offers a full range of information about heart health and disease.

581. Need healthy recipes? Try the American Institute for Cancer Research Recipe Corner at **www.aicr.org/site/Page Server?pagename=dc_rc_home** and 5 A Day Recipes for Fruits and Vegetables at **www.cdc.gov/nccdphp/dnpa/5aday/ recipes/**.

582. Slow Food U.S.A. advocates "living the slow life" by recognizing that food can be a daily pleasure if we make the time for it. It can be especially rewarding if we share meals and meal preparation time with family and friends. Read more about the slow food movement at **www.slowfoodusa.org**.

Online Self-Assessment Tools

583. Try the fat screener and the fruit and vegetable screener, both available free of charge by NutritionQuest at **http:// nutritionquest.com/freetools/index.htm**. These simple quizzes take less than five minutes each to complete, and they provide helpful feedback on recommended saturated fat, fiber, and fruit and vegetable intakes for the reduction of cancer and heart disease risks. (At the time of writing, the quiz does not evaluate trans fat intake.) The researchers who developed these tools also offer a more comprehensive tool that you can order on the site, which produces results similar in accuracy to those obtained through detailed food diaries. The larger quiz takes about half an hour using pencil and paper and costs $15.

584. The NIBBLE nutrition information site sponsored by the University of Massachusetts–Amherst offers a collection of simple quizzes at **www.umass.edu/nibble/ratings/queslist. htm**. It gives feedback on your levels of sugar, sodium, and fat intakes.

585. Try the Rate Your Restaurant Diet at **www.cspinet.org/ nah/quiz/index.html**. This quiz from the Center for Science in the Public Interest is useful for assessing how you do when you are away from home.

Good Reading

586. *Eat, Drink, and Be Healthy: The Harvard Medical School Guide to Healthy Eating,* by Walter Willett (Fireside, 2001).

587. *Fast Food Nation: The Dark Side of the All-American Meal,* by Eric Schlosser (HarperPerennial, 2002).

588. *Fat Land: How Americans Became the Fattest People in the World,* by Greg Critser (Mariner Books, 2004).

589. *Food Politics: How the Food Industry Influences Nutrition and Health,* by Marion Nestle (University of California Press, 2003).

590. *Hungry Planet: What the World Eats,* by Peter Menzel and Faith D'Aluisio (Ten Speed Press, 2005). The authors document in essays and photos what families around the world eat, including a photo of each family with a week's worth of groceries.

591. *Matzoh Ball Gumbo: Culinary Tales of the Jewish South,* by Marcie Cohen Ferris (University of North Carolina at Chapel Hill Press, 2005). Ferris's observations of Jews in the American South help explain how we adapt or adopt new food traditions over time.

Good Eating

593. *Simply Vegan,* 4th edition, by Debra Wasserman and Reed Mangels (Vegetarian Resource Group, 2006).

594. *Kids Can Cook,* by Dorothy Bates (Book Publishing Company, 2000).

595. *The Mediterranean Vegan Kitchen,* by Donna Klein (HP Books, 2001).

596. *The Millennium Cookbook,* by Eric Tucker, John Westerdahl, and Sascha Weiss (Ten Speed Press, 1998).

597. *The Modern Vegetarian Kitchen,* by Peter Berley (Regan Books, 2000).

598. *Munchie Madness: Vegetarian Meals for Teens,* by Dorothy Bates, Bobbie Hinman, and Robert Oser (Book Publishing Company, 2001).

599. *1,000 Vegetarian Recipes,* by Carol Gelles (Macmillan, 1996).

600. *The Teen's Vegetarian Cookbook,* by Judy Krizmanic (Puffin Books, 1999).

601. *Vegetarian Times Complete Cookbook,* by the editors of *Vegetarian Times* (Wiley, 2005).

PART III

The Food Guide and Fat Gram Counter

The food guide that follows lists the trans fat, saturated fat, and combined bad fat content of a sampling of packaged foods in the supermarket as well as foods served at fast-food restaurants. The information was gathered at the time this book was being written, from labels of products on supermarket shelves and from company Web sites.

For that reason, use this food guide to clue you in to foods that may be good or poor choices, but always follow up by reading current labels when you shop. Many food manufacturers are still reformulating their products, so it pays to be diligent about checking labels. You can check company Web sites and in-store brochures for up-to-date nutrition information when you eat at restaurants, too. But precious little information is available at this time about the trans fat content of most restaurant foods.

Whenever the trans fat content of a food was unavailable, I've marked it with a dash on the guide. Several of the fast-food companies don't have trans fat information, and a few of the packaged foods are still without trans fat information on the labels. But I've included as much information as was available in order to make this as comprehensive a list as possible.

You can use the food guide in a few different ways.

◆ Check the trans fat content of your favorite foods. Use the guide to find out whether the foods you eat most often contain trans fats or substantial amounts of saturated fat. If you find that a favorite food contains bad fats, use the guide to identify a healthier substitute.

◆ Construct a shopping list. Use the guide to identify trans-fat-free foods and foods low in total bad fat in various food categories. Again, double-check nutrition labels at the store and compare products to find the best choices.

◆ Push for more healthy choices in stores. Store managers are often receptive to ordering products they don't already stock if they think you and others will buy them. In some cases the store may ask you to buy a carton or a case of the product.

This food guide does not contain an exhaustive list of foods; stores now carry more than forty thousand items, and many of them come on and off the market each year. Others are being reformulated as food companies work to keep up with the demand for foods free of trans fat. In addition to a sampling of information from fast-food restaurants, the guide includes only packaged products bearing nutrition facts labels. Fresh meats and produce don't have nutritional labels and aren't included, but if you would like complete nutrition information about these and other foods not listed, go to the United States Department of Agriculture National Nutrient Database, which is available free at www.nal.usda.gov/fnic/foodcomp/search/.

As I've said elsewhere in this book, but it bears repeating, that when you find the amount of bad fat in a product, pay particular attention to the serving size noted on the label. If it is smaller than what you typically eat, multiply the number of grams of bad fat by the number of servings you will *actually* eat to get a more accurate view of how much bad fat you're likely to get. This is important because amounts shown on food labels can be deceiving. Many foods appear to contain very little bad fat because their listed serving sizes are so much smaller than what people actually eat.

Cookies are a great example. Many brands contain a few grams of bad fat per serving. But let's say their idea of one serving is two small cookies. You and I are both likely to eat two to three times that number at one sitting. In doing so, we're getting substantially more bad fat than what appears on the food label. Factor that reality in when you make decisions about which products to buy and eat.

Use the information in this book—and the food guide that follows—to educate and inform your food choices and help you to achieve a healthier diet. My best wishes to you as you begin.

FOOD GUIDE AND FAT GRAM COUNTER

BRAND NAME	PRODUCT NAME	SERVING SIZE	CALORIES PER SERVING	TOTAL FAT (G) PER SERVING	SATURATED FAT (G) PER SERVING	TRANS FAT (G) PER SERVING	SAT + TRANS (G)
Bagels and Muffins							
Pepperidge Farm	Everything Bagels	1 bagel	260	1.5	0.5	0	0.5
Pepperidge Farm	Plain Bagels	1 bagel	260	1.0	0	0	0
Pepperidge Farm	Plain Mini Bagels	1 bagel	110	0.5	0	0	0
SunMaid	Raisin Bread Cinnamon Swirl	1 slice	100	1.5	0.5	0	0.5
Thomas'	Hearty Grains Multi-Grain English Muffins	1 muffin (57 g)	150	1.5	0	0	0
Thomas'	Hearty Grains 100% Whole Wheat Bagels	1 bagel (104 g)	270	2.0	1.0	0	1.0
Thomas'	New York Style Bagels Everything	1 bagel	300	4.0	1.0	0	1.0
Thomas'	New York Style Bagels Plain	1 bagel	290	2.0	0.5	0	0.5
Thomas'	Original English Muffins	1 muffin	120	1.0	0	0	0
Bread							
Arnold's	100% Whole Wheat	1 slice (90 g)	70	1	0	0	0
Arnold's	Country Classic Oatnut	1 slice (38 g)	110	2	0	0	0
Arnold's	Dutch Country 100% Whole Wheat	1 slice (38 g)	90	1	0	0	0
Arnold's	Dutch Country Butter Split Top	1 slice (35 g)	90	1	0	0	0
Arnold's	Dutch Country Multigrain	1 slice (35 g)	90	1	0	0	0
Arnold's	Dutch Country Soft Potato	1 slice (35 g)	90	1	0	0	0
Arnold's	Raisin Cinnamon	1 slice (32 g)	100	2	1	0	1
Arnold's	Real Jewish Rye, Seedless	1 slice (30 g)	90	1.5	0	0	0
Arnold's	Whole Grain Classics 7 Grain	1 slice (38 g)	100	1	0	0	0
Brownberry	Natural Health Nut	1 slice	100	2.5	0	0	0
Brownberry	Natural Wheat	1 slice	100	1.5	0	0	0

Brand	Product	Serving					
King's Hawaiian	Original	½ inch middle slice	190	4	1.5	0.5	2
King's Hawaiian	Original Rolls	1 roll (28 g)	90	2	1	0	1
Mediterranean	Pita Bread	1 piece (79 g)	190	1.5	0	n/a	n/a
Nature's Own	100% Whole Wheat Whole Grain	1 slice	50	1.0	0	0	0
Nature's Own	Double Fiber Wheat	1 slice	40	1.0	0	0	0
Nature's Own	Honey Wheat	1 slice	60	0.5	0	0	0
Nature's Own	Sugar Free Whole Grain Wheat	1 slice	50	1.0	0	0	0
Nature's Own	White Wheat	1 slice	50	1.0	0	0	0
Nature's Own	Hamburger Butter Buns	1 bun	140	2.5	1.5	0	1.5
Nature's Own	Hamburger Honey Wheat Buns	1 bun	130	1.5	1	0	1
Nature's Own	White Wheat Hot Dog Buns	1 bun	80	1.5	0	0	0
Pepperidge Farm	Carb Style Soft 100% Whole Wheat	1 slice (26 g)	60	1.5	0	0	0
Pepperidge Farm	Crunchy Oat	1 slice (43 g)	120	1.5	0.5	0	0.5
Pepperidge Farm	Farmhouse 12 Grain	1 slice (43 g)	110	2	0.5	0	0.5
Pepperidge Farm	Harvest 7 Grain	1 slice (43 g)	110	1.5	0.5	0	0.5
Pepperidge Farm	Hearty White	1 slice (43 g)	120	1.5	0.5	0	0.5
Pepperidge Farm	Soft Hoagie Rolls	1 roll (68 g)	210	6	2.5	0	2.5
Pepperidge Farm	Whole Grain Swirl	1 slice (38 g)	110	2.5	0.5	0	0.5
Rudi's Organic Bakery	Grain & Flax Bread	1 slice (40 g)	100	2	0	0	0
Rudi's Organic Bakery	Multi Grain Wheat Bread	1 slice (43 g)	110	1	0	0	0
Rudi's Organic Bakery	Sliced Colorado Cracked Wheat	1 slice (43 g)	110	1.5	0	0	0
Rudi's Organic Bakery	Sliced Honey Sweet Whole Wheat	1 slice (43 g)	110	1	0	0	0
Rudi's Organic Bakery	Spelt Bread	1 slice (41 g)	100	1.5	0	0	0
Rudi's Organic Bakery	Wheat & Oat Bread	1 slice (40 g)	90	1	0	0	0
Rudi's Organic Bakery	Wheat Hot Dog Rolls	1 bun (57 g)	150	1.5	0	0	0

BRAND NAME	PRODUCT NAME	SERVING SIZE	CALORIES PER SERVING	TOTAL FAT (G) PER SERVING	SATURATED FAT (G) PER SERVING	TRANS FAT (G) PER SERVING	SAT + TRANS (G)
Bread, Refrigerated							
Pillsbury	Buttermilk Grands	1 biscuit	190	8	3	3	6
Pillsbury	Cinnamon Rolls with Icing	1 roll	150	5	1.5	2	3.5
Pillsbury	Crescent Big & Flaky Dinner Rolls	1 roll	180	10	2.5	2.5	5
Pillsbury	Golden Layers Buttermilk Biscuits	1 biscuit	110	4.5	1	1.5	2.5
Bread, Frozen							
Cole's	Texas Toast	1 slice	170	9	1.5	2	3.5
Pepperidge Farm	Texas Toast	1 slice	150	7	2	1	3
Pillsbury	Oven Baked Biscuits Flaky Layers	1 biscuit	170	8	2	3	5
Pillsbury	Oven Baked Southern Style	1 biscuit	180	9	2.5	4	6.5
Cereals, Cold							
General Mills	Apple Cinnamon Cheerios	¾ cup	120	1.5	0	0	0
General Mills	Cheerios	1 cup	110	2	0	0	0
General Mills	Chex Rice	1¼ cups	120	0.5	0	0	0
General Mills	Cinnamon Toast Crunch	¾ cup	130	3.5	0.5	0	0.5
General Mills	Honey Nut Cheerios	¾ cup	110	1.5	0	0	0
General Mills	Multi Grain Cheerios	1 cup	110	1	0	0	0
General Mills	Raisin Nut Bran	¾ cup	200	3.5	0.5	0.5	1
General Mills	Total	¾ cup	100	0.5	0	0	0
General Mills	Total Raisin Bran	1 cup	170	1	0	0	0
Kellogg's	All Bran	⅓ cup	70	1	0	0	0
Kellogg's	Cracklin Oat Bran	¾ cup	200	7	3	0	3
Kellogg's	Fruit Loops	1 cup	120	1	0.5	0	0.5

Kellogg's	Mini Wheat Frosted	24 biscuits	200	1	0	0	0
Kellogg's	Raisin Bran	1 cup	190	1.5	0	0	0
Kretschmer	Wheat Germ	1/4 cup	30	n/a	0	0	n/a
Post	Bran Flakes	3/4 cup	100	0.5	0	0	0
Post	Grape-Nuts Cereal	1/2 cup	200	1	0	0	0
Post	Grape-Nuts Flakes	3/4 cup	110	1	0	0	0
Post	Honey Bunches of Oats Cereal	3/4 cup	120	1.5	0	0	0
Post	Honeynut Shredded Wheat	1 cup	200	1.5	0	0	0
Post	Raisin Bran	1 cup	190	1	0	0	0
Post	Select Blueberry Morning	1¼ cups	230	3	0	0	0
Post	Select Cranberry Almond Crunch	1 cup	220	3	0	0	0
Post	Shredded Wheat	1 cup	170	1	0	0	0
Quaker	Life Cereal	3/4 cup	120	1.5	0	0	0

Cereals, Hot

Maypo	Maypo Instant	1/2 cup	170	2	0	0	0
Maypo	Vermont Style Oat Cereal	1/3 cup	180	2	0	0	0
Quaker	Instant Oatmeal Cinnamon Roll	1 packet	160	2	0.5	0.5	0.5
Quaker	Instant Oatmeal Dinosaur Eggs	1 packet	200	4	2	2	2
Quaker	Instant Oatmeal Maple Brown Sugar	1 packet	160	2	0	0	0
Quaker	Old Fashioned Oats	1/2 cup	150	3	0.5	0.5	0.5
Quaker	Quick Oats	1/2 cup	150	3	0.5	0.5	0.5
Wheatena	Cereal	1/3 cup	160	1	0	0	0

Cereal Bars

General Mills	Honey Nut Cheerios Milk 'n Cereal Bars	1 bar	160	4	1.5	1	2.5
General Mills	Honey Nut Cheerios Milk 'n Cereal Bars Cinnamon Toast Crunch	1 bar	180	4	1.5	1	2.5

BRAND NAME	PRODUCT NAME	SERVING SIZE	CALORIES PER SERVING	TOTAL FAT (G) PER SERVING	SATURATED FAT (G) PER SERVING	TRANS FAT (G) PER SERVING	SAT + TRANS (G)
General Mills	Honey Nut Cheerios Milk 'n Cereal Bars Coco Puffs	1 bar	160	4	1.5	1	2.5
Health Valley	Strawberry Cobbler Cereal Bars	1 bar	130	2	0	0	0
Kellogg's	Nutri-Grain Cereal Bars Blueberry	1 bar	140	3	0.5	n/a	n/a
Kellogg's	Nutri-Grain Cereal Bars Cherry	1 bar	140	3	0.5	0	0.5
Kellogg's	Nutri-Grain Cereal Bars Raspberry	1 bar	140	3	0.5	0	0.5
Kellogg's	Rice Krispies Treats Original	1 bar	90	2.5	1	0	1
Kellogg's	Rice Krispies Treats Split Stix Chocolatey	1 bar	130	5	3.5	0	3.5
Quaker	Breakfast Bites Apple Crisp	1 pouch	140	2.5	0	0.5	0.5
Quaker	Breakfast Bites Strawberry	1 pouch	140	3	0	0.5	0.5
Quaker	Breakfast Cookies Apple Cinnamon	1 cookie	170	4.5	1.5	0	1.5
Quaker	Breakfast Cookies Oatmeal Raisin	1 cookie	180	4.5	1.5	0	1.5
Breakfast Drinks							
Nestlé	Carnation Instant Breakfast Chocolate	1 packet	130	1	0	0	0
Toaster Pastries							
Kellogg's	Pop-Tart Apple/Cinnamon	1 pastry	210	6	3	0	3
Kellogg's	Pop-Tart Blueberry	1 pastry	210	6	3	0	3
Kellogg's	Pop-Tart Brown Sugar Cinnamon	1 pastry	210	8	4	0	4
Kellogg's	Pop-Tart Frosted Blueberry	1 pastry	200	5	1	0	1
Kellogg's	Pop-Tart Frosted Cherry	1 pastry	200	5	1	n/a	n/a
Kellogg's	Pop-Tart Frosted Chocolate Fudge	1 pastry	200	5	2.5	0	2.5
Kellogg's	Pop-Tart Frosted Cinnamon Brown Sugar	1 pastry	210	7	3.5	0	3.5
Kellogg's	Pop-Tart Frosted Smores	1 pastry	200	5	2.5	0	2.5

Brand	Item	Serving					
Kellogg's	Pop-Tart Frosted Strawberry	1 pastry	200	5	2.5	0	2.5
Kellogg's	Pop-Tart Strawberry	1 pastry	220	6	1.5	n/a	n/a
Kellogg's	Pop-Tart Strawberry Milkshake	1 pastry	200	6	1.5	0	1.5

Frozen Breakfast Items

Brand	Item	Serving					
Aunt Jemima	Buttermilk Pancakes	3	210	3.5	1	0	1
Jimmy Dean	Biscuit Sandwich Sausage	1 sandwich	350	23	8	3	11
Jimmy Dean	Breakfast Skillets Southwestern Style	¼ package	220	12	4.5	0.5	5
Jimmy Dean	Croissant Sandwich Ham & Cheese	1 sandwich	300	17	5	3.5	8.5
Jimmy Dean	Croissant Sandwich Sausage, Egg & Cheese	1 sandwich	450	33	10	4	14
Kellogg's	Eggo Chocolate Chip Waffles	2	200	6	1.5	2	3.5
Kellogg's	Eggo Cinnamon Toast Waffles	3 sets of 4	270	8	2	2.5	4.5
Kellogg's	Eggo French Toaster Sticks Cinnamon	2 pieces	220	6	1	1.5	2.5
Kellogg's	Eggo Homestyle Waffles	2	190	6	1.5	2	3.5
Kellogg's	Eggo Toaster Swirlz Cinnamon Roll Minis	1 set of 4	120	3	0.5	1	1.5
Morning Star Farms	Bacon Strips	2 strips	60	4.5	1.5	0	1.5
Morning Star Farms	Sausage Links	2 links	80	3	0.5	0	0.5
Morning Star Farms	Sausage Patties	1 pattie	80	3	0.5	0	0.5
Pillsbury	Buttermilk Pancakes	3	240	4	1	1	2
Pillsbury	Toaster Scrambles Cheese, Eggs & Sausage	1 pastry	180	12	3.5	n/a	n/a
Pillsbury	Toaster Strudle Apple	1 pastry	190	9	2	2	4
Van's	Organic Original Waffles	2	190	4.5	0	0	0

Spreads

Brand	Item	Serving					
Benecol	Light Spread	1 tbsp	50	5	0.5	0	0.5
Benecol	Spread	1 tbsp	70	8	1	0	1

BRAND NAME	PRODUCT NAME	SERVING SIZE	CALORIES PER SERVING	TOTAL FAT (G) PER SERVING	SATURATED FAT (G) PER SERVING	TRANS FAT (G) PER SERVING	SAT + TRANS (G)
Blue Bonnett	Spread (stick)	1 tbsp	80	9	2	1.5	3.5
Brummel & Brown	Creamy Fruit Spread	1 tbsp	50	4	1	0	1
Brummel & Brown	Spread with Yogurt	1 tbsp	45	5	1	0	1
Canoleo	Soft	1 tbsp	100	11	2	0	2
Earth Balance	Buttery Spread	1 tbsp	100	11	3.5	n/a	n/a
Fleischman's	Original Margarine	1 tbsp	100	11	2	2	4
Fleischman's	Original Spread	1 tbsp	70	8	1.5	0	1.5
I Can't Believe It's Not Butter	Light	1 tbsp	50	5	1	0	1
I Can't Believe It's Not Butter	Original	1 tbsp	90	10	2	2.5	4.5
Kraft	Philadelphia Light Cream Cheese Spread	2 tbsps	60	4.5	3	0	3
Kraft	Philadelphia Original Cream Cheese	1 ounce	100	10	6	0	6
Kraft	Philadelphia Regular Cream Cheese Spread	2 tbsps	90	9	5	0	5
Land O' Lakes	Light Butter with Canola Oil	1 tbsp	50	5	2	0	2
Land O' Lakes	Margarine	1 tbsp	100	11	2	2.5	4.5
Land O' Lakes	Whipped Butter	1 tbsp	50	6	3.5	0	3.5
Parkay	Original Spread	1 tbsp	60	7	1.5	0	1.5
Parkay	Original Spread (stick)	1 tbsp	90	10	2	1.5	3.5
Promise	Light Spread	1 tbsp	45	5	1	0	1
Shedd's Spread	Country Crock	1 tbsp	60	7	1.5	0.5	2
Shedd's Spread	Country Crock Spreadable Sticks	1 tbsp	80	8	1.5	2	3.5
Shedd's Spread	Country Crock Whipped Easy Squeeze	1 tbsp	60	7	1	0	1
Smart Balance	Buttery Spread	1 tbsp	80	9	2.5	0	2.5
Smart Beat	Smart Squeeze	1 tbsp	5	0	0	0	0

Salad Dressings

Avo Classic	Guacamole	2 tbsps	50	4	0.5	0	0.5
Charley's	Honey French	2 tbsps	60	1	0	0.4	0.4
Charley's	Honey Mustard	2 tbsps	176	17	3	0.3	3.3
Charley's	Ranch	2 tbsps	100	10	2	0.5	2.5
Marie's	Chunky Blue Cheese	2 tbsps	170	19	3.5	0	3.5
Marie's	Creamy Ranch	2 tbsps	180	19	3	0	3
T. Marzetti	Asian Ginger	2 tbsps	120	12	2	0	2
T. Marzetti	Chunky Blue Cheese	2 tbsps	150	15	3	0	3
T. Marzetti	Classic Ranch	2 tbsps	160	17	2.5	0	2.5

Condiments

A1	Steak House Marinade Cajun	1 tbsp	25	0	0	0	0
A1	Steak House Marinade Classic	1 tbsp	15	0	0	0	0
Chi-Chi's	Fiesta Salsa Medium	2 tbsps	10	0	0	0	0
Consorzio All Natural	Jamaican Jerk 10-Minute Marinade	1 tbsp	10	0	0	n/a	n/a
Consorzio All Natural	Tropical Grill 10-Minute Marinade	1 tbsp	40	3	0	n/a	n/a
Hellmann's	Real Mayonnaise	1 tbsp	90	10	1.5	0	1.5
Herdez	Salsa Verde Mild	2 tbsps	10	0	0	0	0
KC Masterpiece	Golden Honey Dijon Marinade	1 tbsp	40	0.5	n/a	n/a	n/a
Ken's Steak House	Herb & Garlic Marinade & Sauce	1 tbsp	20	1	0	0	0
Ken's Steak House	Honey Teriyaki Marinade & Sauce	1 tbsp	25	0	0	0	0
Kraft	Miracle Whip Dressing	1 tbsp	40	3.5	0.5	0	0.5
Kraft	Miracle Whip Light Dressing	1 tbsp	25	1.5	0	0	0
Kraft	Original Barbecue Sauce	2 tbsps	40	0	0	0	0
Kraft	Real Mayonnaise	1 tbsp	100	11	1.5	0	1.5
Nasoya	Nayonnaise Sandwich Spread	1 tbsp	35	3.5	0.5	n/a	n/a

BRAND NAME	PRODUCT NAME	SERVING SIZE	CALORIES PER SERVING	TOTAL FAT (G) PER SERVING	SATURATED FAT (G) PER SERVING	TRANS FAT (G) PER SERVING	SAT + TRANS (G)
Newman's Own	Tequila Lime Mild Salsa	2 tbsps	15	0	0	0	0
Ortega	Salsa & Cheese	2 tbsps	90	8	2	0	2
Pace	Chunky Salsa Mild	2 tbsps	10	0	0	0	0
Taco Bell Home Originals	Salsa con Queso	2 tbsps	40	3	0.5	0	0.5
Meals, Frozen							
Amy's	Cheese Pizza	⅓ pizza	310	12	4	0	4
Amy's	Mediterranean Pizza	⅓ pizza	360	15	4.5	0	4.5
Banquet	Beef Pot Pie	1 pie	450	27	11	0.5	11.5
Banquet	Fried Chicken Meal	1 meal	450	20	5	1	6
Banquet	Mexican Style Enchilada Combo Meal	1 meal	400	15	4.5	1	5.5
Boston Market	Beef Pot Roast	1 package	460	19	6	1	7
Boston Market	Beef Sirloin & Noodles	1 package	470	12	4	0.5	4.5
Boston Market	Macaroni & Cheese	½ cup	320	9	4	0	4
Boston Market	Meatloaf with Homestyle Mashed Potatoes & Gravy	1 package	670	39	15	2	17
Boston Market	Pot Pie Turkey	1 cup	560	38	15	0.5	15.5
California Pizza Kitchen	Crispy Thin Crust Margherita	⅓ pizza	300	13	5	0.5	5.5
California Pizza Kitchen	Crispy Thin Crust Sicilian	⅓ pizza	310	14	5	0.5	5.5
California Pizza Kitchen	Crispy Thin Crust White Pizza	⅓ pizza	290	12	6	1	7
DiGiorno	Cheese Stuffed Crust Supreme Pizza	⅙ pizza	350	16	7	0	7
Freschetta	Hand-Tossed Style 4-Meat Pizza	⅙ pizza	340	13	6	0	6
Freschetta	Hand-Tossed Style Pepperoni	⅙ pizza	360	15	7	0	7
Gorton's	Fish Sticks	6 sticks	250	14	3.5	0	3.5

Brand	Product	Serving	Calories				
Gorton's	Premium Fillets Flounder	1 fillet	220	12	2.5	0	2.5
Gorton's	Shrimp Bowl Fried Rice	1 bowl	350	2.5	0.5	0	0.5
Gorton's	Tender's Original Batter	3½ pieces	270	15	3	0	3
Healthy Choice	Mushroom Roasted Beef	1 meal	280	8	3	0	3
Healthy Choice	Salisbury Steak	1 meal	350	8	3.5	0	3.5
Healthy Choice	Sweet and Sour Chicken	1 meal	350	9	3	0	3
Healthy Choice	Sweet Bourbon Steak	1 meal	310	7	2.5	0	2.5
Hungry Man	Classic Fried Chicken	1 package	960	45	10	n/a	n/a
Hungry Man	Salisbury Steak	1 package	490	18	4.5	n/a	n/a
Hungry Man	XXL Backyard Barbeque	1 package	1160	48	18	n/a	n/a
Marie Callender's	Country Fried Chicken & Gravy	1 meal	670	37	14	n/a	n/a
Marie Callender's	Grilled Chicken Alfredo Bake	1 meal	610	37	16	n/a	n/a
Marie Callender's	Meatloaf and Gravy	1 meal	560	31	14	n/a	n/a
Marie Callender's	Swedish Meatballs	1 meal	580	30	14	n/a	n/a
Mrs. Paul's	Crunchy Fish Sticks	6 sticks	230	12	2	2	4
Mrs. Paul's	Lightly Breaded Flounder Fillets	1 fillet	150	7	3.5	0	3.5
Stouffer's	Chicken Lasagna	1 cup	330	15	3.5	0	3.5
Stouffer's	Corner Bistro Sesame Chicken	1 package	510	15	2.5	0	2.5
Stouffer's	Green Pepper Steak	1 package	310	8	2.5	0	2.5
Stouffer's	Grilled Chicken Teriyaki	1 package	300	3.5	1	0	1
Stouffer's	Grilled Lemon Pepper Chicken	1 package	250	7	2	0	2
Stouffer's	Lasagna with Meat & Sauce	1 cup	290	12	5	0	5
Stouffer's	Lean Cuisine Deluxe Cheddar Potato	1 package	260	7	3.5	0	3.5
Stouffer's	Lean Cuisine Hunan Beef & Broccoli	1 package	230	4	1.5	0	1.5
Stouffer's	Lean Cuisine Lemongrass Chicken	1 package	250	6	3.5	0	3.5
Stouffer's	Lean Cuisine Pork with Cherry Sauce	1 package	250	4.5	2	0	2
Stouffer's	Macaroni & Cheese	1 cup	390	20	9	n/a	n/a
Stouffer's	Meatloaf Dinner	1 package	590	32	12	0	12

BRAND NAME	PRODUCT NAME	SERVING SIZE	CALORIES PER SERVING	TOTAL FAT (G) PER SERVING	SATURATED FAT (G) PER SERVING	TRANS FAT (G) PER SERVING	SAT + TRANS (G)
Stouffer's	Meatloaf in Gravy	1 loaf & gravy	220	14	6	0	6
Stouffer's	Roast Turkey Breast Dinner	1 package	440	16	5	0	5
Stouffer's	Spaghetti with Meat Sauce	1 package	350	12	4	0	4
Stouffer's	Stuffed Peppers	1 pepper & sauce	180	7	2.5	0	2.5
Stouffer's	White Meat Chicken Pot Pie	½ pie	580	35	15	0	15
Swanson	Boneless Fried Chicken	1 package	520	22	5	n/a	n/a
Swanson	Chicken Pot Pie	1 package	410	23	10	n/a	n/a
Swanson	Fried Chicken Strips	1 package	640	30	7	n/a	n/a
Swanson	Roasted Carved Turkey	1 package	430	17	4	n/a	n/a
Tony's	Original Crust Cheese	⅓ pizza	380	16	9	0	9
Tony's	Original Crust Pepperoni Pizza	⅓ pizza	420	21	10	2	12
Tyson	Chicken Quick Breast Tenders	5 pieces	220	13	3	0	3
Tyson	Chicken Quick Nuggets	5 pieces	280	18	4	0	4
Tyson	Honey BBQ Chicken Wings	3 pieces	250	15	3.5	0	3.5
Weight Watchers	Smart Ones Beef Pot Roast	1 package	170	5	2	0	2
Weight Watchers	Smart Ones Home-Style Chicken	1 package	230	9	3.5	0	3.5
Weight Watchers	Smart Ones Slow-Roasted Turkey Breast	1 package	210	7	2	0	2
Weight Watchers	Smart Ones Three Cheese Ziti Marinara	1 package	290	7	2.5	0	2.5

Meals, Packaged Mixes

BRAND NAME	PRODUCT NAME	SERVING SIZE	CALORIES PER SERVING	TOTAL FAT (G) PER SERVING	SATURATED FAT (G) PER SERVING	TRANS FAT (G) PER SERVING	SAT + TRANS (G)
Betty Crocker	Au Gratin Real Potatoes	⅔ cup prepared	150	6	1.5	1	2.5
Betty Crocker	Bacon Cheeseburger	1 cup prepared	380	18	7	n/a	n/a

Brand	Product	Serving					
Betty Crocker	Cheesy Scalloped Potatoes	½ cup prepared	150	6	1.5	1	2.5
Betty Crocker	Chicken Helper Cheesy Chicken Enchilada	1 cup prepared	320	7	2	1	3
Betty Crocker	Complete Meals Chicken & Buttermilk Biscuits	⅕ package	280	11	4	3	7
Betty Crocker	Complete Meals Three Cheese Chicken	⅕ package	260	10	2.5	1.5	4
Betty Crocker	Crunchy Taco	1 cup prepared	330	14	5	1.5	6.5
Betty Crocker	Hamburger Helper Cheesy Baked Potato	1 cup prepared	310	14	5	1.5	6.5
Betty Crocker	Hamburger Helper Cheesy Jambalaya	1 cup prepared	330	14	5	1	6
Betty Crocker	Hamburger Helper Chili Cheese	1 cup prepared	340	13	5	1.5	6.5
Betty Crocker	Hamburger Helper Philly Cheesesteak	1 cup prepared	330	17	6	1.5	7.5
Betty Crocker	Microwave Singles Cheeseburger Macaroni	1 pouch	220	6	2	1.5	3.5
Betty Crocker	Microwave Singles Cheesy Beef Taco	1 pouch	220	6	2	1.5	3.5
Betty Crocker	Microwave Singles Stroganoff	1 pouch	190	4	1	1	2
Betty Crocker	Roasted Garlic and Cheddar Mashed Potatoes	½ cup prepared	160	8	2	1.5	3.5
Betty Crocker	Tuna Helper Creamy Broccoli	1 cup prepared	290	11	3	2.5	5.5
Betty Crocker	Tuna Helper Creamy Pasta	1 cup prepared	290	13	3.5	3	6.5
Old El Paso	8 Flour Tortillas for Burritos	1	130	4	1	1	2
Old El Paso	8 Taco Salad Shells	1 shell	110	6	1	2	3
Old El Paso	12 Flour Tortillas for Soft Tacos and Fajitas	2 tortillas	160	4.5	1	1.5	2.5

BRAND NAME	PRODUCT NAME	SERVING SIZE	CALORIES PER SERVING	TOTAL FAT (G) PER SERVING	SATURATED FAT (G) PER SERVING	TRANS FAT (G) PER SERVING	SAT + TRANS (G)
Old El Paso	12 Taco Shells	3	150	7	1.5	2.5	4
Old El Paso	12 White Corn Taco Shells	3	150	6	1.5	2.5	4
Old El Paso	Soft Taco Bake Dinner Kit (prepared with lean ground beef)	1 serving (¼ box)	430	23	8	4	12
Old El Paso	Soft Taco Dinner Kit (prepared with lean ground beef)	1 serving (⅕ box)	380	18	7	2	9
Old El Paso	Super Stuffer 10 Taco Shells	2 shells	170	8	1.5	3	4.5
Old El Paso	Taco Dinner Kit (prepared with lean ground beef)	1 serving (⅙ box)	280	15	5	2.5	7.5
Ortega	Taco Kit	1 serving (⅙ box)	150	5	1	n/a	n/a
Meals, Ready-to-Eat							
Armour	LunchMakers Chicken Nuggets	1 package	180	5	1	0	1
Kraft	South Beach Diet Southwestern Style Chicken Wraps	1 package	250	10	5	0	5
Kraft	South Beach Diet Turkey & Bacon Club Wraps	1 package	250	13	4.5	0	4.5
Oscar Mayer	Lunchables All-Star Hotdogs	1 package	400	13	7	0	7
Oscar Mayer	Lunchables BBQ Chicken Shakeups	1 package	210	6	2	0	2
Oscar Mayer	Lunchables Bologna & American Stackers	1 package	480	20	9	0.5	9.5
Oscar Mayer	Lunchables Chicken Dunks	1 package	310	6	2	0	2
Oscar Mayer	Lunchables Ham & Cheddar w/ crackers	1 package	340	18	9	1	10
Oscar Mayer	Lunchables Mega Chicken Strips	1 package	570	15	4	1	5
Oscar Mayer	Lunchables Mega Deep Dish Pizza Extra Cheesy	1 package	710	20	9	0.5	9.5

Brand	Product	Serving	Cal	Fat	Sat	Trans	Total
Oscar Mayer	Lunchables Nachos	1 package	380	21	6	0	6
Oscar Mayer	Lunchables Pizza & Treatza	1 package	460	10	4.5	0	4.5
Oscar Mayer	Lunchables Pizza Extra Cheesy	1 package	310	10	4.5	0	4.5
Oscar Mayer	Lunchables Tacos	1 package	460	12	5	0	5
Oscar Mayer	Lunchables Turkey & Cheddar Stackers	1 package	380	13	6	0.5	6.5

Pasta Sauces

Brand	Product	Serving	Cal	Fat	Sat	Trans	Total
Classico	Cabernet Marinara with Herbs	½ cup	60	2	0	0	0
Classico	Four Cheese Alfredo	¼ cup	80	7	4	0	4
Classico	Sun-Dried Tomato Sauce	½ cup	80	3	1	0	1
Hunt's	Garlic & Herb Spaghetti Sauce	½ cup	40	0.5	0	0	0
Hunt's	Organic Roasted Garlic Pasta Sauce	½ cup	50	0	0	0	0
Hunt's	Original Style Traditional	½ cup	50	0.5	0	0	0
Newman's Own	Italian Sausage & Peppers Pasta Sauce	½ cup	90	4	1	0	1
Newman's Own	Sockarooni	½ cup	70	2	0	0	0
Newman's Own	Vodka Sauce Pasta Sauce	½ cup	110	5	1.5	0	1.5
Prego	Chunky Garden Pasta Sauce	½ cup	110	3.5	1	0	1
Prego	Organic Tomato and Basil Pasta Sauce	½ cup	90	2.5	0	0	0
Prego	Three Cheese Pasta Sauce	½ cup	90	1.5	0	0	0
Ragu	Carb Options Double Cheddar Sauce	¼ cup	90	8	2.5	0	2.5
Ragu	Cheesy Classic Alfredo	¼ cup	110	10	3.5	0	3.5
Ragu	Rich & Meaty Mama's Meat Sauce	½ cup	110	5	1.5	0	1.5

Sides, Frozen

Brand	Product	Serving	Cal	Fat	Sat	Trans	Total
Bright Harvest	Scalloped Sweet Potatoes	⅓ cup	170	7	3	1	4
Bright Harvest	Sweet Potato Casserole	⅓ cup	300	14	2.5	1	3.5
Ore-Ida	Country Inn Creations Peppers & Onion Hash Browns	1 cup	90	4	0.5	0.5	1

BRAND NAME	PRODUCT NAME	SERVING SIZE	CALORIES PER SERVING	TOTAL FAT (G) PER SERVING	SATURATED FAT (G) PER SERVING	TRANS FAT (G) PER SERVING	SAT + TRANS (G)
Ore-Ida	Country Inn Creations Savory Seasoned Hash Browns	1 cup	110	4.5	0.5	0.5	1
Ore-Ida	Extra Crispy Fast Food Fries	27 pieces	160	6	1.5	2	3.5
Ore-Ida	Extra Crispy Golden Crinkles	14 pieces	170	7	1.5	2	3.5
Ore-Ida	Texas Crispers! Potato Wedges	8 pieces	140	6	1.5	2	3.5
Ore-Ida	Zesties!	12 pieces	140	5	1	2	3
Poppers	Cheddar Cheese Jalapeños	3 pieces	210	13	4	0.5	4.5
Stouffer's	Corn Soufflé	½ cup	150	5	1	0	1
Stouffer's	Creamed Spinach	½ package	200	16	7	n/a	n/a
Stouffer's	Harvest Apples	⅔ cup	190	2.5	0.5	n/a	n/a
TGI Friday's	Cheddar & Bacon Potato Skins	3 pieces	210	12	4	1	5

Sides, Refrigerated

BRAND NAME	PRODUCT NAME	SERVING SIZE	CALORIES PER SERVING	TOTAL FAT (G) PER SERVING	SATURATED FAT (G) PER SERVING	TRANS FAT (G) PER SERVING	SAT + TRANS (G)
Simply Potatoes	Garlic Mashed Potatoes	⅔ cup	170	10	5	1	6
Simply Potatoes	Sour Cream & Chive Mashed Potatoes	⅔ cup	170	10	5	1	6

Crackers

BRAND NAME	PRODUCT NAME	SERVING SIZE	CALORIES PER SERVING	TOTAL FAT (G) PER SERVING	SATURATED FAT (G) PER SERVING	TRANS FAT (G) PER SERVING	SAT + TRANS (G)
Austin	Cheese Crackers with Cheddar Cheese	1 package	210	10	2	4	6
Austin	Cheese Crackers with Cheddar Jack Cheese	1 package	200	11	2.5	4.5	7
Austin	Cheese Crackers with Peanut Butter	1 package	200	10	1.5	2	3.5
Austin	Grilled Cheese Flavored Cracker Sandwiches	1 package	200	10	2	4	6
Austin	Mega Stuffed Cheese Crackers with Peanut Butter	1 package	240	13	2	2	4
Austin	PB&J Flavored Cracker Sandwiches	1 package	200	10	2	3.5	5.5
Keebler	Club Crackers	4 crackers	70	3	1	0	1

Keebler	Zesta Wheat	5 crackers	60	1.5	0.5	0.5	1
Lance	Captain's Wafers	6 crackers	200	10	2	0	2
Lance	Cheese on Wheat	6 crackers	190	9	1.5	0	1.5
Lance	Nip-Chee	6 crackers	190	9	1.5	0	1.5
Nabisco	Better Cheddars Baked Snack Crackers	22 crackers	150	8	2	0.5	2.5
Nabisco	Cheese Nips	19 crackers	130	4.5	1	0	1
Nabisco	Chicken in a Biskit Baked Snack Crackers	12 crackers	170	10	2	0.5	2.5
Nabisco	Garden Herb Triscuit	6 crackers	120	4	0.5	0	0.5
Nabisco	Mixers Cheddar Snack Mix	½ cup	130	4.5	1	n/a	n/a
Nabisco	Original Premium Saltine Crackers	5 crackers	60	1.5	0	0	0
Nabisco	Ritzbits Cheese	13 sandwiches	150	9	3.5	0	3.5
Nabisco	Triscuit Original	6 crackers	120	4.5	0.5	0	0.5
Nonni's	Garlic Italian Toast	5 pieces	120	4	1	n/a	n/a
Pepperidge Farm	Cheddar Goldfish	55 pieces	140	5	1	0	1
Pepperidge Farm	Goldfish	55 pieces	140	5	1	0	1
Pepperidge Farm	Goldfish Colors	55 pieces	140	5	1	0	1
Stella D'Oro	Original Breadstick	1 breadstick	40	1	0	0	0
Sunshine	Cheez It	27 crackers	160	8	2	0	2
Sunshine	Cheez It Twisterz Cheddar	17 crackers	140	6	2.5	0	2.5
Sunshine	Twisterz Cool Ranch & Cheddar	17 crackers	140	6	2.5	0	2.5
Wheat Thins	Harvest Five Grain Baked Snack Crackers	13 crackers	130	3.5	1	0	1
Wheat Thins	Multigrain Wheat Thin	17 crackers	130	4.5	0.5	0	0.5
Wheat Thins	Wheat Thin Chips	13 chips	130	4	0.5	0	0.5

Microwave Popcorn

Jiffy Pop	Butter Flavored Popcorn	About 1 cup	140	7	1.5	3	4.5
Jolly Time	Blast O Butter Microwave Popcorn	3½ cups	150	12	3	4	7
Jolly Time	Healthy Pop Kettle Corn	4 cups	90	2	0	0	0

BRAND NAME	PRODUCT NAME	SERVING SIZE	CALORIES PER SERVING	TOTAL FAT (G) PER SERVING	SATURATED FAT (G) PER SERVING	TRANS FAT (G) PER SERVING	SAT + TRANS (G)
Orville Redenbacher's	Gourmet Popping Corn Butter	5 cups	170	12	6	0	6
Orville Redenbacher's	Movie Theater Butter Microwave Popcorn	1 cup	35	2.5	1	0	1
Pop Secret	Homestyle Popcorn	4 cups	170	12	3	5	8
Pop Secret	Light Butter	3 tbsp (6 cups)	120	6	1.5	2	3.5
Pop Secret	Movie Theater Butter Microwave Popcorn	1 cup	40	3	0.5	1	1.5
Snack Chips							
Cape Cod	40% Reduced Fat	19 chips	130	6	1.5	0	1.5
Cape Cod	Beachside BBQ Chips	19 chips	150	9	2.5	0	2.5
Cape Cod	Jalapeño Cheddar	18 chips	140	8	2	0	2
Cape Cod	Regular Chips	19 chips	150	8	2	0	2
Cape Cod	Sea Salt & Vinegar	18 chips	150	8	2	0	2
Lay's	Stax Hidden Valley Ranch	12 crisps	150	9	2.5	0	2.5
Lay's	Classic Chip	20 chips	150	10	3	0	3
Lay's	KC Masterpiece	11 chips	120	3	0	0	0
Lay's	Salt & Vinegar	17 chips	150	10	3	0	3
Lay's	Wavy Original	11 chips	150	10	2.5	0	2.5
Pringles	CheezUms	14 crisps	150	11	3	0	3
Pringles	Original	14 crisps	160	11	3	0	3
Ruffles	Baked Ruffles Original	10 crisps	120	3	0	0	0
Snyder's of Hanover	Butter Snaps	24 pretzels	120	1	0	0	0
Snyder's of Hanover	Olde Tyme Pretzel	28 sticks	120	1	0	0	0
Snyder's of Hanover	Pretzel Rod	3 pretzels	120	1	0	0	0

Snyder's of Hanover	Sourdough Special	1	120	1	0	0	0
Snyder's of Hanover	White Corn Tortilla Chips	13 chips	140	4.5	0	0	0
Snyder's of Hanover	Yellow Corn Tortilla Chips	13 chips	140	4.5	0	0	0
Utz	Cheddar & Sour Cream Potato Chips	About 20 chips (1 oz)	150	9	2	0	2
Utz	Honey BBQ Potato Chips	About 20 chips (1 oz)	150	9	2	0	2
Utz	No Salt Potato Chips	About 20 chips (1 oz)	150	9	2	0	2
Utz	Potato Chips	About 20 chips (1 oz)	150	9	2	0	2
Utz	Salt & Vinegar Potato Chips	About 20 chips (1 oz)	150	9	2	0	2
Wise	Cheez Doodles Crunchy	½ cup	150	9	2.5	0	2.5
Wise	Cheez Doodles Puffed	23 pieces	150	8	2	0	2
Wise	Regular Chips	16 chips	150	10	3	0	3
Wise	Ridgies Chips	15 chips	150	10	3	0	3
Energy Bars							
Atkins	Advantage Chocolate Peanut Butter Bar	1 bar	240	12	6	n/a	n/a
Atkins	Advantage S'mores Bar	1 bar	220	10	5	n/a	n/a
Atkins	Endulge Caramel Nut Chew	1 bar	140	7	3.5	0	3.5
Atkins	Endulge Chocolate Covered Coconut	1 bar	180	12	9	0	9
Balance	Gold Crunch Chocolate Mint Cookie	1 bar	210	6	4	0	4
Balance	Gold Crunch Cookies n Creme	1 bar	210	6	4	0	4
Balance	Gold Rocky Road	1 bar	210	7	4	0	4
Cliff Bar	Chocolate Chip	1 bar	250	5	2	0	2
Cliff Bar	Cranberry Apple Cherry	1 bar	230	2.5	0.5	0	0.5
Cliff Bar	Crunchy Peanut Butter	1 bar	250	6	1.5	0	1.5

BRAND NAME	PRODUCT NAME	SERVING SIZE	CALORIES PER SERVING	TOTAL FAT (G) PER SERVING	SATURATED FAT (G) PER SERVING	TRANS FAT (G) PER SERVING	SAT + TRANS (G)
Kashi	Go Lean Cookies & Cream	1 bar	290	6	4	n/a	n/a
Kashi	Go Lean Oatmeal Raisin Cookie	1 bar	280	5	3	0	3
Kashi	Go Lean Peanut Butter & Chocolate	1 bar	290	6	4.5	0	4.5
Luna	Dulce de Leche	1 bar	180	3	1	0	1
Luna	Key Lime Pie	1 bar	180	4	3	0	3
Luna	S'mores	1 bar	180	5	3	0	3
Power Bar	Performance Peanut Butter	1 bar	240	3.5	0.5	0	0.5
Power Bar	Protein Plus Chocolate Crisp	1 bar	290	6	3.5	0	3.5
Power Bar	Triple Threat Chocolate Caramel Fushion	1 bar	230	8	4.5	0	4.5
Power Bar	Triple Threat Chocolate Peanut Butter Crisp	1 bar	220	5	2	0	2
Slim-Fast	Optima Meal Bar Caramel Crispy Peanut	1 bar	220	6	4	0	4
Slim-Fast	Optima Meal Bar Milk Chocolate Peanut	1 bar	220	5	3	0	3
Slim-Fast	Optima Meal Bar Strawberry Cheesecake	1 bar	220	6	4	0	4
Snickers	Marathon Energy Bar Chewy Chocolate Peanut	1 bar	220	7	2.5	0	2.5
Snickers	Marathon Energy Bar Low Carb Peanut Butter	1 bar	170	6	2	0	2
Snickers	Marathon Energy Bar Multi-Grain Crunch	1 bar	220	7	2.5	0	2.5

Granola Bars

BRAND NAME	PRODUCT NAME	SERVING SIZE	CALORIES PER SERVING	TOTAL FAT (G) PER SERVING	SATURATED FAT (G) PER SERVING	TRANS FAT (G) PER SERVING	SAT + TRANS (G)
Betty Crocker	Fruit Gushers Variety Pack	1 pack	90	1	0	0	0
Cascadian Farm	Organic Chewy Granola Fruit & Nut Bars	1 bar	140	4	0.5	0	0.5
Kashi	Honey Almond Flax Chewy Granola Bars	1 bar	140	5	0.5	0	0.5

Brand	Product	Serving	Calories				
Kashi	Peanut Peanut Butter Chewy Granola Bars	1 bar	130	5	0.5	0	0.5
Kellogg's	Nutri-Grain Yogurt Bars, Strawberry	1 bar	140	3	0.5	0	0.5
Kellogg's	Special K Bar, Strawberry	1 bar	90	1.5	1	0	1
Nature Valley	Chewy Trail Mix Fruit & Nut	1 bar	140	4	0.5	0	0.5
Nature Valley	Crunchy Granola Bar, Roast Almond	2 bars	190	7	1	0	1
Nature Valley	Crunchy Granola Bar, Peanut Butter	2 bars	180	7	1	0	1
Nature Valley	Granola Bar Variety	2 bars	180	6	0	0	0
Nature Valley	Healthy Heart Chewy Oatmeal Raisin	1 bar	150	2	0.5	0	0.5
Nature Valley	Sweet & Salty Nut Almond	1 bar	160	7	2	0	2
Quaker	Chewy Cinnamon Sugar	1 bar	110	2	0.5	0	0.5
Quaker	Chewy Dipps Peanut Butter	1 bar	150	7	3	0	3
Quaker	Chewy Peanut Butter Chocolate Chunk	1 bar	120	3.5	1	0	1
Quaker	Chewy S'mores Lowfat	1 bar	110	2	0.5	0	0.5
Quaker	Crunchy Granola Bars Oats, Nuts & Honey	2 bars	130	4	0.5	0	0.5
Sunbelt	Chewy Oatmeal/Honey	1 bar	130	5	3	0	3

Appetizers, Snacks, and Sandwiches—Frozen

Brand	Product	Serving	Calories				
Boca	Meatless Burgers Roasted Onion	1 burger	70	1	0	0	0
Croissant Pockets	Meatballs & Mozzarella	1 piece	330	15	5	n/a	n/a
Croissant Pockets	Turkey Bacon Club	1 piece	320	15	6	n/a	n/a
Farm Rich	Breaded Onion Petals	10 pieces	200	12	2	1	3
Hooters	Buffalo Shrimp	7 shrimp	280	13	2.5	2	4.5
Hooters	Buffalo Style Chicken Strips	3 ounces	160	6	1	0.5	1.5
Hooters	Chicken Wings	3 ounces	230	15	3.5	0.5	4
Hot Pockets	Chicken Fajita	1 piece	290	11	4	n/a	n/a
Hot Pockets	Hearty Sized Biscuits	1 piece	280	13	6	0	6
Hot Pockets	Subs, Meatballs & Mozzarella	1 piece	390	14	5	n/a	n/a
Hot Pockets	Subs, Pepperoni Pizza	1 piece	410	16	6	n/a	n/a

BRAND NAME	PRODUCT NAME	SERVING SIZE	CALORIES PER SERVING	TOTAL FAT (G) PER SERVING	SATURATED FAT (G) PER SERVING	TRANS FAT (G) PER SERVING	SAT + TRANS (G)
Morning Star Farms	Chik Patties	1 pattie	170	7	1	0	1
Morning Star Farms	Chik'n Nuggets	4 nuggets	190	7	1	0	1
Morning Star Farms	Chik'n Tenders Honey Mustard	2 pieces	190	7	1	0	1
Morning Star Farms	Corn Dogs	1 corn dog	150	4	0.5	0	0.5
Morning Star Farms	Veggie Burgers Garden Veggie Patties	1 pattie	100	2.5	0.5	0	0.5
Morning Star Farms	Veggie Burgers Grillers Prime	1 burger	170	9	1	0	1
Morning Star Farms	Veggie Dogs	1 link	80	0.5	0	0	0
TGI Friday's	Cheddar & Bacon Potato Skins	3 pieces	210	12	4	1	5
TGI Friday's	Mexican Style Queso Dip	2 tbsps	50	3.5	2	n/a	n/a
TGI Friday's	Mozzarella Sticks	1 piece	100	6	2	0	2
TGI Friday's	Southwestern Egg Rolls	1 piece	210	8	2.5	0.5	3
TGI Friday's	Steak Quesadilla Rolls	2 pieces	200	8	2	0.5	2.5
TGI Friday's	Sweet & Smoky Popcorn Chicken	5 pieces	250	8	1.5	1	2.5

Sandwich Spreads

BRAND NAME	PRODUCT NAME	SERVING SIZE	CALORIES PER SERVING	TOTAL FAT (G) PER SERVING	SATURATED FAT (G) PER SERVING	TRANS FAT (G) PER SERVING	SAT + TRANS (G)
Dickinson's	Lime Curd	1 tbsps	60	1	0.5	0	0.5
Durkee-Mower	Marshmallow Fluff	2 tbsps	60	0	0	0	0
Ferrero	Nutella Hazelnut Spread	2 tbsps	200	11	2	0	2
Jif	Creamy Peanut Butter	2 tbsps	190	16	3	0	3
Jif	Reduced Fat Creamy Peanut Butter	2 tbsps	190	12	2.5	0	2.5
Peter Pan	Creamy Peanut Butter	2 tbsps	190	17	3.5	0	3.5
Peter Pan	Plus Creamy Peanut Butter	2 tbsps	190	16	3	0	3
Skippy	Creamy Peanut Butter	2 tbsps	190	16	3	0	3
Smucker's	Goober Grape Peanut Butter & Jelly Stripes	3 tbsps	240	13	2.5	0	2.5
Smucker's	Natural Peanut Butter Chunky	2 tbsps	210	16	2.5	0	2.5

Cakes & Doughnuts

Brand	Item	Serving					
BlueBird	6 Pecan Spins	1	100	4	1.5	0	1.5
Dolly	Danish Rollers	2	200	8	1.5	0	1.5
Entenmann's	Cinnamon Swirl Bun	1	320	14	6	0	6
Entenmann's	Crumb Coffee Cake	⅛ cake	260	12	5	0	5
Entenmann's	Frosted Chocolate Donuts	1	310	26	16	0	16
Entenmann's	Raspberry Danish Twist	⅛ danish	220	11	5	0	5
Entenmann's	20 Softees Cocos Locos Coconut Donuts	4	320	15	9	0	9
Entenmann's	20 Softees Frosted Donuts	3	230	14	9	0	9
Entenmann's	20 Softees Plain Donuts	4	250	14	7	0	7
Entenmann's	20 Softees Powdered Donuts	4	240	11	2.5	n/a	n/a
Entenmann's	Enten-mini's Caramel & Crème Squares	2	270	11	8	0	8
Entenmann's	Enten-mini's Carrot Cake	1	160	7	1.5	0	1.5
Entenmann's	Enten-mini's Chocolate ½ Rounds	1	140	7	4	0	4
Entenmann's	Glazed Popems	4 pieces	220	10	5	0	5
Entenmann's	Little Bites Chocolate Chip Mini Muffins	1 pouch	210	10	2.5	0	2.5
Entenmann's	Little Bites Fudge Brownies	1 pouch	270	15	4	0	4
Entenmann's	Little Bites Rainbow Chip Blondies	1 pouch	260	11	3.5	0	3.5
Entenmann's	Ultimate Chocolate Lovers Variety Donuts 8 Pack Devil's-Food Crumb Donuts	1	260	13	7	0	7
Entenmann's	Ultimate Chocolate Lovers Variety Donuts 8 Pack Frosted Devil's-Food Donuts	1	310	19	6	0	6
Entenmann's	Ultimate Chocolate Lovers Variety Donuts 8 Pack Rich-Frosted Donuts	1	280	19	12	0	12
Entenmann's	Ultimate Chocolate Lovers Variety Donuts 8 Pack Rich-Frosted Donuts with White Drizzle	1	290	19	12	0	12

BRAND NAME	PRODUCT NAME	SERVING SIZE	CALORIES PER SERVING	TOTAL FAT (G) PER SERVING	SATURATED FAT (G) PER SERVING	TRANS FAT (G) PER SERVING	SAT + TRANS (G)
Entenmann's	Ultimate Super Cinnamons	½ bun	320	13	6	0	6
Hostess	Brownie Bites	1 pouch	290	14	4	3.5	7.5
Hostess	Cup Cakes	1	180	6	2.5	0	2.5
Hostess	Frosted Donettes	3	220	13	9	0	9
Hostess	Ho Hos	3	380	17	12	0.5	12.5
Hostess	Mini Muffins Banana Walnut	1 pouch	230	14	2	0	2
Hostess	Mini Muffins Blueberry	1 pouch	250	13	2.5	0	2.5
Hostess	Powdered Donettes	4	240	12	6	0.5	6.5
Hostess	Suzy Q's	1	220	8	4.5	0	4.5
Hostess	Sweet Rolls Cinnamon	1	210	7	2.5	0	2.5
Hostess	Twinkies	1	150	4.5	2.5	0	2.5
Krispy Kreme	Chocolate Iced Doughnuts	1	250	12	4	3	7
Krispy Kreme	Chocolate Iced Kreme Filled Doughnuts	1	350	20	5	6	11
Krispy Kreme	Mini Crullers Glazed	2	220	15	3.5	5	8.5
Krispy Kreme	Original Glazed	1	200	12	3	4	7
Krispy Kreme	Original Glazed Donut Holes	5 pieces	200	11	3	3.5	6.5
Little Debbie	Boston Creme Rolls	1	270	12	4	2	6
Little Debbie	Devil Cremes Cakes	1	200	9	2	2	4
Little Debbie	Donut Sticks	1	230	14	7	0	7
Little Debbie	Fudge Brownie	1	290	13	3.5	0.5	4
Little Debbie	Fudge Rounds	1	310	12	4.5	0.5	5
Little Debbie	Honey Buns	1	220	12	6	0	6
Little Debbie	Lemon Cupcakes	1	170	7	2	0	2
Little Debbie	Nutty Bars	2	320	20	8	0	8
Little Debbie	Pecan Spinwheels	1	100	4	1	0	1

Brand	Product	Serving					
Little Debbie	Reduced Fat Oatmeal Creme Pies	1	150	2.5	0.5	0	0.5
Little Debbie	Swiss Roll	2	270	12	5	0	5
Little Debbie	Zebra Cakes	2	330	15	8	0	8
Merita	Sweet Sixteen Donuts, Chocolate Frosted	3	260	16	11	0.5	11.5
Merita	Sweet Sixteen Donuts, Sugar	3	230	12	6	1	7
Moon Pie	Chocolate Moon Pie Original	1	152	4.5	3	0	3
Moon Pie	Mini Moon Pie Chocolate	1 package	150	4.5	3	0	3
Moon Pie	Moon Pie Chocolate	1 package	226	5.7	3.5	0	3.5

Cake and Brownie Mixes and Frosting

Brand	Product	Serving					
Betty Crocker	Rich & Creamy Coconut Pecan Frosting	2 tbsps (35 g)	140	7	3	1.5	4.5
Betty Crocker	Rich & Creamy Rainbow Chip Frosting	2 tbsps (34 g)	140	5	2	1.5	3.5
Betty Crocker	Super Moist German Chocolate Cake Mix	1/12 package	270	13	3	0.5	3.5
Betty Crocker	Warm Delights Fudgy Chocolate Chip Cookie Cookie Mix	1 bowl (82 g)	340	11	4.5	1	5.5
Betty Crocker	Warm Delights Molten Caramel Cake Cake Mix	1 bowl (95 g)	360	10	3.5	2	5.5
Duncan Hines	Bakery-Style Cinnamon Swirl Muffins Mix	1 muffin (45 g mix)	200	6	1.5	1	2.5
Duncan Hines	Bakery-Style Wild Maine Blueberry Muffins Mix	1 muffin (45 g mix)	150	4.5	1	1	2
Duncan Hines	Candy Shop Brownies Peanut Butter Cup	1/16 package	170	8	2.5	0.5	3
Duncan Hines	Chocolate Lovers Brownies	1/16 package	170	7	2	0.5	2.5
Duncan Hines	Creamy Home-Style Classic Chocolate Frosting	2 tbsps (35 g)	130	6	1.5	1.5	3

BRAND NAME	PRODUCT NAME	SERVING SIZE	CALORIES PER SERVING	TOTAL FAT (G) PER SERVING	SATURATED FAT (G) PER SERVING	TRANS FAT (G) PER SERVING	SAT + TRANS (G)
Duncan Hines	Creamy Home-Style Lemon Supreme Frosting	2 tbsps (35 g)	140	6	1.5	1.5	3
Duncan Hines	Signature Dessserts Chocolate Silk Torte	1/10 package (63 g)	440	18	5	0.5	5.5
Ghirardelli	Chocolate Walnut Brownies Mix	1 brownie (30 g)	170	5*	1*	1*	2*
Pillsbury	Creamy Supreme Chocolate Fudge Frosting	2 tbsps (35 g)	140	6	1.5	2	3.5
Pillsbury	Creamy Supreme Cream Cheese Frosting	2 tbsps (35 g)	150	6	1.5	2	3.5
Pillsbury	Ultimate Dessert Kit, Cookies 'n Crème	1/9 package (53 g)	270	5*	1.5*	1.5*	3.0*
Pillsbury	Ultimate Muffins, Caramel Apple Streusel	1/12 package (54 g)	270	4.5*	1.5*	1*	2.5*

* Fat content could be higher depending on ingredients added to mix at home.

Cookies

Archway	Apple Oatmeal	1	90	2.5	0.5	1	1.5
Archway	Brownie bars	1	190	7	2.5	1.5	4
Archway	Chocolate Chip	3	160	7	2.5	1.5	4
Archway	Chocolate Sandwich Crème	3	170	8	5	1	6
Archway	Classic Oatmeal	1	110	4	1	1	2
Archway	Coconut Crème	2	190	8	4	1.5	5.5
Archway	Coconut Macaroon	1	80	4.5	4	0	4
Archway	Double Fudge Crème	2	190	9	4	1.5	5.5

Brand	Product						
Archway	Frosty Lemon	1	110	4.5	1.5	1	2.5
Archway	Gingersnap	5	150	5	1	1.5	2.5
Archway	Iced Oatmeal	1	110	4.5	1	1	2
Archway	Oatmeal Classic	1	110	4	1	1	2
Archway	Oatmeal Raisin	2	140	6	1.5	2	3.5
Archway	Oatmeal Raisin Big Batch	1	120	2.5	1	1	2
Archway	Old Fashioned Molasses	1	110	3	0.5	1	1.5
Archway	Pecan Shortbread	2	160	9	2	2.5	4.5
Carr's	Table Water Cracker	5	70	1.5	0.5	0	0.5
Dove	Chocolate Walnut Oasis	1	110	6	3	0	3
Dove	Milk Chocolate Moment	3	160	9	5	0	5
Dove	Mint Chocolate Serenade	3	160	8	5	0	5
Famous Amos	Chocolate Chip	4	140	7	2	2	4
Famous Amos	Chocolate Chip & Pecans	4	150	8	2.5	1.5	4
Keebler	Animal Crackers	10	130	3.5	1	0	1
Keebler	Chips Deluxe Original	1	80	4	1	1.5	2.5
Keebler	Chips Deluxe Peanut Butter Cups	1	90	4.5	2	1.5	3.5
Keebler	Country Style Oatmeal	2	130	6	1.5	2.5	4
Keebler	E.L. Fudge Double Stuffed	2	180	9	2	3.5	5.5
Keebler	Fudge Shoppe Caramel Filled	2	160	8	5	1	6
Keebler	Fudge Shoppe Deluxe Grahams	3	140	7	4.5	1.5	6
Keebler	Fudge Stripes	3	160	7	4	1.5	5.5
Keebler	Sandies Chocolate Chip & Pecan Shortbread	1	80	5	1	1.5	2.5
Keebler	Soft Batch Oatmeal Raisin	1	80	3	0.5	1	1.5
Keebler	Vienna Fingers	2	150	7	1.5	2.5	4
Mrs. Fields	Milk Chocolate Chip	1	160	8	5	0	5
Mrs. Field's	Decadent Chocolate Grahams	1	90	4.5	2.5	0	2.5
Mrs. Field's	Oatmeal Raisin with Nuts	1	150	7	3	0	3

BRAND NAME	PRODUCT NAME	SERVING SIZE	CALORIES PER SERVING	TOTAL FAT (G) PER SERVING	SATURATED FAT (G) PER SERVING	TRANS FAT (G) PER SERVING	SAT + TRANS (G)
Mrs. Field's	White Chunk Macadamia	1	150	8	4.5	0	4.5
Murray	Vanilla Wafer	8	150	6	1.5	2.5	4
Murray	Duplex Cremes	3	130	5	1.5	2	3.5
Murray	Lemon Cremes	3	150	6	1	2	3
Murray	Old Fashioned Ginger Snaps	5	140	4.5	1	1.5	2.5
Murray	Sugar Free Chocolate Chip	3	140	8	2.5	2.5	5
Murray	Sugar Free Double Fudge	3	140	7	2	2	4
Murray	Sugar Free Fudge Dipped Grahams	4	140	8	5	1.5	6.5
Murray	Sugar Free Lemoncream	3	130	7	1.5	2.5	4
Murray	Sugar Free Pecan Shortbread	3	170	11	2.5	3.5	6
Murray	Sugar Free Shortbread Cookies	8	140	6	1.5	2	3.5
Murray	Sugar Wafers	5	160	7	1.5	2.5	4
Murray	Vanilla Cremes	3	140	5	1	2	3
Nabisco	Candy Chips Ahoy	1	80	4	2	0	2
Nabisco	Chewy Chips Ahoy	2	120	6	3	0	3
Nabisco	Chips Ahoy	3	160	8	2.5	0	2.5
Nabisco	Chips Ahoy 100% Whole Grain	3	150	8	2.5	0	2.5
Nabisco	Chips Ahoy Chunky	1	80	4	1.5	0	1.5
Nabisco	Chips Ahoy Soft Baked Chunky	1	120	5	3	0	3
Nabisco	Chips Ahoy White Fudge Chunky	1	80	4	1.5	0	1.5
Nabisco	Chocolate Chewy Chips Ahoy	2	120	6	3	0	3
Nabisco	Chocolate Grahams	8 (2 sheets)	130	3	0.5	1	1.5
Nabisco	Chocolate Teddy Graham	24 pieces	130	4.5	1	0	1
Nabisco	Cinnamon Teddy Graham	24 pieces	130	4	1	0	1

Brand	Product	Serving					
Nabisco	Fig Newtons	2	110	2	0	0	0
Nabisco	Fig Newtons 100% Whole Grain	2	110	2	0.5	0	0.5
Nabisco	Gingersnaps	4	120	2.5	0.5	0	0.5
Nabisco	Graham Cinnamon	4 (1 sheet)	130	3.5	1	0	1
Nabisco	Graham Crackers	8 (2 sheets)	130	3	0.5	0	0.5
Nabisco	Honey Maid Oatmeal	3	150	6	1.5	0	1.5
Nabisco	Nilla Wafer	8	110	2	0	0	0
Nabisco	Nutter Butter	2	130	6	1	n/a	n/a
Nabisco	Oreo Double Stuff	2	140	7	2.5	0	2.5
Nabisco	Pure Milk Chocolate Covered Nutter Butter	1	90	4.5	2	0	2
Nabisco	Pure Milk Chocolate Covered Oreo	1	90	4.5	2.5	0	2.5
Nabisco	SnackWell's Cookie Cakes Black Forest	1	50	0.5	0	0	0
Nabisco	SnackWell's Creme Sandwich	2	110	3	1	0	1
Nabisco	Sugar-Free Oreo	2	100	5	1.5	0	1.5
Nabisco	Teddy Graham Honey	24 pieces	130	4	1	0	1
Pepperidge Farm	Bordeaux Cookie	4	130	5	3.5	0	3.5
Pepperidge Farm	Brussels Cookie	3	150	7	4	0	4
Pepperidge Farm	Butter Chessmen	3	120	5	3	0	3
Pepperidge Farm	Milano Cookie	3	180	10	5	0	5
Pepperidge Farm	Milk Chocolate Macadamia Nut	1	140	8	3.5	0	3.5
Pepperidge Farm	Snickerdoodle	1	140	5	2.5	0	2.5
Stella D'Oro	Original Breadstick	1	40	1	0	0	0

Candy

Brand	Product	Serving					
Dove	Smooth Milk Chocolate	5 pieces (40 g)	220	13	8	0	8
Hershey's	Miniatures	5 pieces (43 g)	230	13	7	0	7

223

BRAND NAME	PRODUCT NAME	SERVING SIZE	CALORIES PER SERVING	TOTAL FAT (G) PER SERVING	SATURATED FAT (G) PER SERVING	TRANS FAT (G) PER SERVING	SAT + TRANS (G)
Kraft	Caramels	5 pieces (40 g)	160	3.5	1	1	2
Lindt	Swiss Bittersweet Fine Dark Chocolate	12 blocks (40 g)	210	13	8	0	8
M&M's	M&M's	¼ cup (42 g)	210	9	6	0	6
Reese's	Peanut Butter Cups	1 piece (15 g)	80	4.5	1.5	0	1.5
Toblerone	Swiss Milk Chocolate with Honey/Almond Nougat	⅓ bar (33 g)	170	10	6	0	6
York	Peppermint Pattie	1 pattie (39 g)	160	3	1.5	0	1.5
Desserts, Frozen or Refrigerated							
Edwards	Banana Cream Pie	⅙ pie	470	27	19	2	21
Edwards	Chocolate Silk Pie	⅛ pie	490	31	17	4	21
Edwards	Key Lime Pie	⅛ pie	450	22	15	1.5	16.5
Mrs. Smith's	Boston Cream Pie	⅒ pie	220	9	2.5	0	2.5
Mrs. Smith's	Cherry Pie	⅛ pie	330	16	7	0	7
Mrs. Smith's	Cinnabon Cinnamon Pecan Coffee Cake	⅛ cake	270	17	3.5	3	6.5
Mrs. Smith's	Hearty Pumpkin Pie	⅛ pie	280	12	2.5	n/a	n/a
Mrs. Smith's	Hearty Pumpkin Spiced Pie	⅛ pie	300	14	6	0	6
Mrs. Smith's	Lemon Meringue	⅛ pie	300	10	2	2.5	4.5
Mrs. Smith's	Mince Pie	⅛ pie	360	16	3	4	7
Mrs. Smith's	Sweet Potato Pie	⅛ pie	350	18	7	0	7

Ice Cream

Brand	Product	Serving					
Pepperidge Farm	3-Layer Cake Chocolate Fudge Stripe	1/8 cake	250	13	3	3.5	6.5
Pepperidge Farm	3-Layer Cake Golden	1/8 cake	250	12	2.5	3.5	6
Pepperidge Farm	Turnovers Apple	1	290	15	4	5	9
Pepperidge Farm	Turnovers Cherry	1	280	15	4	5	9
Sara Lee	All Butter Pound Cake	1/6 cake	300	16	8	1	9
Sara Lee	Pecan Coffee Cake	1/6 cake	190	10	2	2.5	4.5
Ben & Jerry's	Cherry Garcia	1/2 cup	250	14	10	0	10
Ben & Jerry's	Cherry Garcia Low Fat Frozen Yogurt	1/2 cup	170	3	2	0	2
Ben & Jerry's	Chocolate Chip Cookie Dough	1/2 cup	270	15	10	0	10
Ben & Jerry's	Chocolate Fudge Brownie Low Fat Frozen Yogurt	1/2 cup	190	2.5	1.5	0	1.5
Ben & Jerry's	Chubby Hubby	1/2 cup	320	20	11	0	11
Ben & Jerry's	Dublin Mudslide	1/2 cup	270	16	10	0	10
Ben & Jerry's	New York Super Fudge Chunk	1/2 cup	310	20	11	0	11
Ben & Jerry's	Phish Food Frozen Yogurt	1/2 cup	210	4.5	3	0	3
Ben & Jerry's	Vanilla	1/2 cup	240	15	10	0	10
Breyers	Carb Smart Chocolate	1/2 cup	120	8	5	0	5
Breyers	Carb Smart Vanilla	1/2 cup	110	8	5	0	5
Breyers	Cherry Vanilla	1/2 cup	140	6	4	0	4
Breyers	Cookies & Cream	1/2 cup	150	7	5	0	5
Breyers	Extra Creamy Vanilla	1/2 cup	140	7	4.5	0	4.5
Breyers	Light Vanilla	1/2 cup	100	3.5	2	0	2
Breyers	M&M's Vanilla Fudge	1/2 cup	170	10	5	n/a	n/a
Breyers	Natural Vanilla	1/2 cup	140	7	4.5	0	4.5
Breyers	No Sugar Added Triple Chocolate	1/2 cup	110	5	3	0	3
Breyers	No Sugar Added Vanilla	1/2 cup	80	4	2.5	0	2.5

BRAND NAME	PRODUCT NAME	SERVING SIZE	CALORIES PER SERVING	TOTAL FAT (G) PER SERVING	SATURATED FAT (G) PER SERVING	TRANS FAT (G) PER SERVING	SAT + TRANS (G)
Breyers	Peach	½ cup	120	5	3	0	3
Edy's	Grand Butter Pecan	½ cup	170	10	4.5	0	4.5
Edy's	Grand Double Vanilla	½ cup	140	7	4.5	0	4.5
Edy's	Light Coffee	½ cup	105	3.5	2	0	2
Edy's	Light Cookie Dough	½ cup	130	4.5	3	0	3
Edy's	Light Vanilla	½ cup	100	3.5	2	0	2
Edy's	No Sugar Added Mint Chocolate Chips	½ cup	110	4.5	3	0	3
Edy's	No Sugar Added Vanilla	½ cup	90	0	0	0	0
Häagen-Dazs	Caramel Cone	½ cup	320	19	10	0.5	10.5
Häagen-Dazs	Light Dulce de Leche	½ cup	220	7	4.5	0	4.5
Häagen-Dazs	Macadamia Brittle	½ cup	300	20	12	n/a	n/a
Häagen-Dazs	Rum Raisin	½ cup	270	17	10	0.5	10.5
Häagen-Dazs	Sorbet Mango	½ cup	150	0	0	0	0
Häagen-Dazs	Vanilla	½ cup	270	18	11	n/a	n/a
Healthy Choice	Caramel Fudge Brownie	½ cup	120	2	1	n/a	1
Healthy Choice	Cookies 'N Cream	½ cup	120	2	1	n/a	n/a
Healthy Choice	Mint Chocolate Chip	½ cup	110	1.5	1	0	1
Healthy Choice	No Sugar Added Coffee Almond Fudge	½ cup	110	2	1	0	1
Healthy Choice	No Sugar Added Vanilla	½ cup	100	1.5	1	0	1
Healthy Choice	Vanilla	½ cup	110	2	1	n/a	1

Frozen Novelties

Breyers	Carb Smart Almond Bar	1	180	15	10	0	10
Dove	Miniatures	5 pieces	300	20	13	0	13

Brand	Product	Serving					
Dove	Original Vanilla Ice Cream Bars	1	260	17	11	0	11
Edy's	Dibs	26 pieces	390	29	18	0	18
Edy's	Fruit Bars Lime	1	80	0	0	0	0
Edy's	Fruit Bars Whole Fruit	1	80	0	0	0	0
Häagen-Dazs	Brownie Bar	1	360	24	13	n/a	n/a
Häagen-Dazs	Vanilla & Milk Chocolate Bar	1	290	21	14	0	14
Healthy Choice	Premium Sorbet & Cream Bars	1	90	1	0.5	0	0.5
Healthy Choice	Premium Vanilla Sandwiches	1	130	2	1	0	1
Minute Maid	Juice Bars	1	60	0	0	0	0
Nestlé	Crunch Ice Cream Bars	1	220	15	11	0	11
Nestlé	Drumstick	1	340	21	11	0	11
Nestlé	Scooby-Doo Push-Up	1	120	6	3.5	n/a	n/a
Pet	Ice Cream Sandwiches	1	160	5	3	0	3
Popsicle	Fudgsicle Original Fudge Bar	1	70	0	0	0	0
Popsicle	Orange Cherry Grape	1	40	0	0	0	0
Weight Watchers	Giant Chocolate Fudge Ice Cream Bar	1	110	1	0.5	0	0.5
York	Klondike Bars	1	250	17	12	0	12

Piecrusts

Brand	Product	Serving					
Mrs. Smith's	Deep Dish Pie Shells	⅛ pie shell	130	7	3.5	0	3.5
Pillsbury Pet Ritz	Regular Pie Crust	⅛ crust	80	4	1.5	0	1.5
Pepperidge Farm	Puff Pastry Shells	1	190	13	3.5	5	4
Pepperidge Farm	Puff Pastry Sheets	⅙ sheet	170	11	3	4	7
Keebler	Ready Crust Graham	⅛ crust	100	4.5	2	2	4
Keebler	Ready Crust Shortbread	⅙ crust	100	4.5	2	2	4

BRAND NAME	PRODUCT NAME	SERVING SIZE	CALORIES PER SERVING	TOTAL FAT (G) PER SERVING	SATURATED FAT (G) PER SERVING	TRANS FAT (G) PER SERVING	SAT + TRANS (G)
Shortening							
Crisco	All-Vegetable Shortening	1 tbsp (12 g)	110	12	3	1.5	4.5
Crisco	All-Vegetable Shortening	1 tbsp (12 g)	110	12	3	1.5	4.5
Crisco	0 Grams Trans Fat Per Serving All-Vegetable Shortening	1 tbsp (12 g)	110	12	3	0	3
Fast Food							
ARBYS							
Breakfast Foods	Plain Biscuit	73 g	230	12	3	not listed	n/a
	Bacon Biscuit	86 g	300	17	5	n/l	n/a
	Ham Biscuit	116 g	270	13	3.5	n/l	n/a
	Sausage Biscuit	113 g	390	27	9	n/l	n/a
	Bacon'n Egg Croissant	125 g	410	26	12	n/l	n/a
	Ham'n Cheese Croissant	118 g	350	19	11	n/l	n/a
	Sausage'n Egg Croissant	152 g	510	36	15	n/l	n/a
	Sourdough Ham, Egg'n Swiss	237 g	450	23	8	n/l	n/a
	Sourdough Bacon, Egg'n Swiss	211 g	500	29	10	n/l	n/a
	Sourdough Egg'n Cheese	144 g	330	16	6	n/l	n/a
Roast Beef	Big Montana	309 g	590	29	14	n/l	n/a
Sandwiches	Giant Roast Beef	224 g	450	19	9	n/l	n/a
	Regular Roast Beef	154 g	320	13	6	n/l	n/a
	Beef'n'Cheddar	195 g	440	21	7	n/l	n/a
	Super Roast Beef	230 g	440	19	7	n/l	n/a
	Junior Roast Beef	125 g	270	9	4	n/l	n/a

Other Sandwiches

Chicken Breast Fillet	233 g	500	25	4	n/l	n/a
Chicken Bacon'n Swiss	209 g	550	27	7	n/l	n/a
Chicken Fingers 4 Pack	192 g	640	38	8	n/l	n/a
Chicken Fingers Combo	320 g	1050	60	11	n/l	n/a
Roast Chicken Club	228 g	470	25	7	n/l	n/a

Market Fresh Sandwiches

Market Fresh Roast Turkey, Ranch & Bacon	379 g	830	38	10	n/l	n/a
Market Fresh Ultimate BLT	293 g	780	46	9	n/l	n/a
Market Fresh Roast Beef & Swiss	357 g	780	39	12	n/l	n/a
Market Fresh Roast Ham & Swiss	357 g	700	31	7	n/l	n/a
Market Fresh Roast Turkey & Swiss	357 g	720	27	6	n/l	n/a
Market Fresh Chicken Salad	322 g	770	38	9	n/l	n/a

Market Fresh Wraps

Ultimate BLT Wrap	254 g	650	47	11	n/l	n/a
Roast Turkey, Ranch & Bacon Wrap	338 g	710	39	11	n/l	n/a
Southwest Chicken Wrap	259 g	550	30	9	n/l	n/a
Chicken Club Wrap	321 g	680	38	14	n/l	n/a

Market Fresh Salads (no dressing)

Martha's Vineyard	291 g	250	8	4.5	n/l	n/a
Santa Fe	328 g	520	29	9	n/l	n/a
Chicken Club Salad	405 g	530	33	10	n/l	n/a

Premium Potatoes

Curly Fries (small)	106 g	340	18	3	n/l	n/a
Homestyle Fries (small)	113 g	300	13	2	n/l	n/a
Potato Cakes (2)	100 g	250	15	2	n/l	n/a

BRAND NAME	PRODUCT NAME	SERVING SIZE	CALORIES PER SERVING	TOTAL FAT (G) PER SERVING	SATURATED FAT (G) PER SERVING	TRANS FAT (G) PER SERVING	SAT + TRANS (G)
Sidekickers	Jalapeño Bites (regular)	110 g	310	19	7	n/l	n/a
	Mozzarella Sticks (regular)	137 g	430	23	10	n/l	n/a
	Onion Petals (regular)	113 g	330	19	3	n/l	n/a
Desserts	Apple Turnover (no icing)	89 g	250	10	3	n/l	n/a
	Cherry Turnover (no icing)	89 g	250	10	3	n/l	n/a
	Gourmet Chocolate Cookie	45 g	200	10	6	n/l	n/a
BOJANGLES							
Cajun Style Chicken	Breast	n/l	278	17	n/l	n/l	n/a
	Leg	n/l	264	16	n/l	n/l	n/a
	Thigh	n/l	310	23	n/l	n/l	n/a
	Wing	n/l	355	25	n/l	n/l	n/a
Southern Style Chicken	Breast	n/l	261	16	n/l	n/l	n/a
	Leg	n/l	254	15	n/l	n/l	n/a
	Thigh	n/l	308	21	n/l	n/l	n/a
	Wing	n/l	337	21	n/l	n/l	n/a
Sweet Biscuits	Bo Berry	n/l	220	10	3	n/l	n/a
	Cinnamon	n/l	320	18	4	n/l	n/a
Biscuit Sandwiches	Biscuit (plain)	n/l	243	12	3	n/l	n/a
	Bacon	n/l	290	17	5	n/l	n/a
	Bacon, Egg & Cheese	n/l	550	42	14	n/l	n/a
	Cajun Filet	n/l	454	21	6	n/l	n/a

Country Ham	n/l	270	15	4	n/l	n/a
Egg	n/l	400	30	6	n/l	n/a
Sausage	n/l	350	23	7	n/l	n/a
Smoked Sausage	n/l	380	26	9	n/l	n/a
Steak	n/l	649	49	13	n/l	n/a
Sandwiches						
Cajun Fillet (no mayo)	n/l	337	11	5	n/l	n/a
Grilled Fillet (no mayo)	n/l	235	5	3	n/l	n/a
Cajun Fillet with mayo	n/l	437	22	7	n/l	n/a
Grilled Fillet with mayo	n/l	335	16	5	n/l	n/a
Individual Fixin's						
Botato Rounds	n/l	235	11	4	n/l	n/a
Cajun Pintos	n/l	110	0	0	n/l	n/a
Marinated Cole Slaw	n/l	136	3	0	n/l	n/a
Corn on the Cob	n/l	140	2	0	n/l	n/a
Dirty Rice	n/l	166	6	2	n/l	n/a
Green Beans	n/l	25	0	0	n/l	n/a
Macaroni & Cheese	n/l	198	14	5	n/l	n/a
Potatoes without gravy	n/l	80	1	0	n/l	n/a
Seasoned Fries	n/l	344	19	5	n/l	n/a
Snacks						
Chicken Supremes	n/l	337	16	6	n/l	n/a
Buffalo Bites	n/l	180	5	2	n/l	n/a
BURGER KING						
Breakfast Items						
Croissan'wich with Egg & Cheese	115 g	300	17	6	2	8
Croissan'wich with Sausage & Cheese	106 g	370	25	9	2	11
French Toast Sticks, 5 sticks	112 g	390	20	4.5	4.5	9
Hash Brown Rounds	75 g	230	15	4	5	9

BRAND NAME	PRODUCT NAME	SERVING SIZE	CALORIES PER SERVING	TOTAL FAT (G) PER SERVING	SATURATED FAT (G) PER SERVING	TRANS FAT (G) PER SERVING	SAT + TRANS (G)
	Enormous Omelet Sandwich	266 g	740	46	16	1	17
	Croissan'wich with Sausage, Egg & Cheese	159 g	470	32	11	2.5	13.5
	Croissan'wich with Bacon, Egg & Cheese	122 g	340	20	7	2	9
	Croissan'wich with Ham, Egg & Cheese	149 g	340	18	6	2	8
Meat Sandwiches	Hamburger	121 g	290	12	4.5	0.5	5
	Cheeseburger	133 g	330	16	7	0.5	7.5
	Bacon Cheeseburger	141 g	370	19	8	0.5	8.5
	The Angus Steak Burger	290 g	560	22	8	1.5	9.5
	Original Whopper Sandwich	290 g	670	39	11	1.5	12.5
Chicken and Fish	Chicken Tenders (5 pieces)	77 g	210	12	3	2	5
	Tendercrisp Chicken Sandwich	300 g	780	43	8	4	12
	BK Big Fish Sandwich	250 g	630	30	6	2.5	8.5
	Tendergrill Chicken Sandwich	258 g	450	10	2	0	2
	BK Chicken Fries 6 piece with Buffalo Sauce	114 g	340	24	4.5	3	7.5
Salads and Veggies	BK Veggie Burger	215 g	420	16	2.5	0	2.5
	Tendercrisp Garden Salad (without dressing)	385 g	410	21	6	3.5	9.5
	Tendercrisp Caesar Salad (without dressing)	327 g	400	21	6	3.5	9.5
	Side Garden Salad (without dressing)	106 g	20	0	0	0	0
	Tendergrill Garden Salad	357 g	230	8	3	0	3
	Tendergrill Caesar Salad	299 g	220	8	3	0	3

Treats

Dutch Apple Pie	108 g	300	13	3	3	6
Hershey's Sundae Pie	79 g	300	18	10	1.5	11.5
Vanilla Shake (small)	298 g	400	15	10	0	10
Chocolate Shake (small)	284 g	410	13	8	0	8
Strawberry Shake (small)	284 g	410	13	8	0	8
Icee Coca-Cola® (small)	242 g	110	0	0	0	0
Icee Cherry (small)	242 g	110	0	0	0	0

KFC

Salads and More

Caesar Side Salad	76 g	50	3	2	0	2
Crispy BLT Salad	360 g	350	17	4.5	3	7.5
Crispy Caesar Salad	315 g	370	19	7	3.5	10.5
House Side Salad	83 g	15	0	0	0	0
Mashed Potato Bowl with Gravy	490 g	690	31	9	4.5	13.5
Mashed Potato Bowl with HBBQ	490 g	710	29	8	4.5	12.5
Rice Bowl with Gravy	472 g	770	25	8	4	12
Roasted BLT Salad	347 g	210	7	2.5	0	2.5
Roasted Caesar Salad	301 g	220	9	4.5	0.5	5
Tender Roast Fillet Meal	321 g	360	7	2	0.5	2.5

Sandwiches and Twisters

Crispy Twister	252 g	670	38	7	3	10
Double Crunch Sandwich	213 g	520	28	6	3	9
Honey BBQ KFC Snacker	101 g	220	3.5	1	0	1
Honey BBQ Sandwich	147 g	300	6	1	0.5	1.5
KFC Snacker	119 g	320	16	3	1.5	4.5
Oven Roasted Twister	269 g	520	23	4	0	4
Triple Crunch Sandwich	262 g	640	34	7	4.5	11.5

BRAND NAME	PRODUCT NAME	SERVING SIZE	CALORIES PER SERVING	TOTAL FAT (G) PER SERVING	SATURATED FAT (G) PER SERVING	TRANS FAT (G) PER SERVING	SAT + TRANS (G)
Chicken	Extra Crispy Chicken Breast	162 g	460	28	8	4.5	12.5
	Extra Crispy Chicken Drumstick	60 g	160	10	2.5	1.5	4
	Extra Crispy Chicken Thigh	114 g	370	26	7	3	10
	Extra Crispy Chicken Whole Wing	52 g	190	12	4	2	6
	Hot and Spicy Chicken Breast	179 g	460	27	8	4.5	12.5
	Hot and Spicy Chicken Drumstick	60 g	150	9	2.5	1.5	4
	Hot and Spicy Chicken Thigh	128 g	400	28	8	3	11
	Hot and Spicy Chicken Whole Wing	55 g	180	11	3	2	5
	Original Recipe Chicken Original Recipe Chicken Breast with skin or breading	161 g	380	19	6	2.5	8.5
	Original Recipe Chicken Original Recipe Chicken Breast w/o skin or breading	108 g	140	3	1	0	1
	Original Recipe Chicken Original Recipe Chicken Drumstick	59 g	140	8	2	1	3
	Original Recipe Chicken Original Recipe Chicken Thigh	126 g	360	25	7	1.5	8.5
	Original Recipe Chicken Original Recipe Chicken Whole Wing	47 g	150	9	2.5	1	3.5
Miscellaneous	Crispy Strips (3 pieces)	151 g	400	24	5	4.5	9.5
	Popcorn Chicken (Individual)	114 g	380	21	5	4.5	9.5
	Pot Pie	423 g	770	40	15	0	15
Buffalo Wings	Boneless Fiery Buffalo Wings	211 g	520	25	4.5	4.5	9
	Boneless HBBQ Wings	213 g	510	24	4.5	4.5	9

Category	Item	Serving	Calories				
	Boneless Sweet & Spicy Wings	203 g	540	24	4.5	4.5	9
	Fiery Buffalo Wings	171 g	440	27	7	3.5	10.5
	Honey BBQ Wings	157 g	540	33	7	0	7
	Hot Wings	134 g	450	29	6	0	6
	Sweet & Spicy Wings	158 g	460	26	7	3.5	10.5
Bread	Biscuit	57 g	190	10	2	0	2
Side Items	BBQ Baked Beans	136 g	230	1	1	0	1
	Cole Slaw	130 g	190	11	2	0	2
	Corn on the Cob, small	82 g	70	1.5	0.5	0	0.5
	Green Beans	96 g	50	1.5	0	0	0
	Mac and Cheese	136 g	130	6	2	0	2
	Mashed Potatoes and Gravy	136 g	130	4.5	1	0.5	1.5
	Potato Salad	128 g	180	9	1.5	0	1.5
	Potato Wedges	102 g	240	12	3	4	7
	Seasoned Rice	99 g	150	1	0	0	0
Desserts	Apple Pie Minis (3)	114 g	400	22	5	0	5
	Apple Pie Slice	108 g	270	9	2	0	2
	Double Chocolate Chip Cake	76 g	400	29	5	0	5
	Lemon Meringue Pie Slice	92 g	310	11	5	0	5
	Lil' Bucket Chocolate Crème	113 g	270	13	8	0	8
	Lil' Bucket Fudge Brownie	99 g	270	9	4	0	4
	Lil' Bucket Lemon Crème	127 g	400	14	7	0	7
	Lil' Bucket Strawberry Short Cake	99 g	200	6	4	0	4
	Pecan Pie Slice	95 g	370	15	2.5	0	2.5

BRAND NAME PRODUCT NAME	SERVING SIZE	CALORIES PER SERVING	TOTAL FAT (G) PER SERVING	SATURATED FAT (G) PER SERVING	TRANS FAT (G) PER SERVING	SAT + TRANS (G)
McDonald's						
Breakfast Items						
Egg McMuffin	4.9 oz (138 g)	290	11	4.5	0	4.5
Sausage McMuffin	4 oz (114 g)	370	21	9	0.5	9.5
Sausage McMuffin with Egg	5.8 oz (164 g)	450	26	10	0.5	10.5
English Muffin	2 oz (57 g)	150	2	1	0	1
Bacon, Egg & Cheese Biscuit	5.1 oz (145 g)	440	24	8	5	13
Sausage Biscuit with Egg	5.7 oz (162 g)	500	32	10	5	15
Sausage Biscuit	4 oz (112 g)	410	26	8	5	13
Biscuit	2.4 oz (69 g)	240	11	2.5	5	7.5
Bacon, Egg & Cheese McGriddles	5.9 oz (168 g)	450	21	7	1.5	8.5
Sausage, Egg & Cheese McGriddles	7 oz (199 g)	560	32	11	1.5	12.5
Sausage McGriddles	4.7 oz (135 g)	420	22	7	1.5	8.5
Big Breakfast	9.4 oz (266 g)	730	46	14	7	21
Deluxe Breakfast	15.3 oz (437 g)	1220	60	17	11	28
Sausage Burrito	4 oz (113 g)	300	16	6	1	7
Hotcakes and Sausage	9.2 oz (264 g)	770	33	9	4	13
Hotcakes (2 pats margarine & syrup)	7.6 oz (221 g)	600	17	4	4	8
Sausage Patty	1.5 oz (43 g)	170	15	6	0	6
Scrambled Eggs (2)	3.6 oz (101 g)	180	11	4	0	4
Hash Browns	1.9 oz (53 g)	140	8	1.5	2	3.5
Warm Cinnamon Roll	3.7 oz (105 g)	420	18	4.5	4.5	9
Deluxe Warm Cinnamon Roll	5.7 oz (162 g)	590	24	7	6	13
Grape Jam	0.5 oz (14 g)	35	0	0	0	0
Strawberry Preserves	0.5 oz (14 g)	35	0	0	0	0

Sandwiches

Hamburger	3.7 oz (105 g)	260	9	3.5	0.5	4
Cheeseburger	4.2 oz (119 g)	310	12	6	1	7
Double Cheeseburger	6.1 oz (173 g)	460	23	11	1.5	12.5
Quarter Pounder	6.1 oz (171 g)	420	18	7	1	8
Quarter Pounder with Cheese	7 oz (199 g)	510	25	12	1.5	13.5
Double Quarter Pounder with Cheese	9.9 oz (280 g)	730	40	19	3	22
Big Mac	7.8 oz (219 g)	560	30	10	1.5	11.5
Big N' Tasty	8.2 oz (232 g)	470	23	8	1.5	9.5
Big N' Tasty with Cheese	8.7 oz (247 g)	520	26	10	1.5	11.5
Filet-O-Fish	5 oz (141 g)	400	18	4	1	5
McChicken	5.2 oz (147 g)	370	16	3.5	1	4.5
Hot 'n Spicy McChicken	5.1 oz (146 g)	380	17	3.5	1	4.5
Premium Grilled Chicken Classic Sandwich	8 oz (229 g)	420	9	2	0	2
Premium Crispy Chicken Classic Sandwich	8.2 oz (232 g)	500	16	3	1.5	4.5
Premium Grilled Chicken Club Sandwich	9.4 oz (268 g)	590	22	8	0	8
Premium Crispy Chicken Club Sandwich	9.6 oz (272 g)	680	29	9	1.5	10.5
Premium Grilled Chicken Ranch BLT Sandwich	8.5 oz (242 g)	490	13	4	0	4
Premium Crispy Chicken Ranch BLT Sandwich	8.6 oz (245 g)	580	20	5	1.5	6.5

French Fries

Small French Fries	2.6 oz (74 g)	230	11	2	2.5	4.5

Chicken Nuggets

Chicken McNuggets (4 piece)	2.3 oz (64 g)	170	10	2	1	3

Salads

Bacon Ranch Salad with Grilled Chicken	11.2 oz (320 g)	260	9	4	0	4
Bacon Ranch Salad with Crispy Chicken	11.4 oz (323 g)	340	16	5	1.5	6.5
Bacon Ranch Salad (without chicken)	7.9 oz (223 g)	140	7	3.5	0	3.5
Caesar Salad with Grilled Chicken	10.9 oz (310 g)	220	6	3	0	3
Caesar Salad with Crispy Chicken	11 oz (313 g)	300	13	4	1.5	5.5

BRAND NAME	PRODUCT NAME	SERVING SIZE	CALORIES PER SERVING	TOTAL FAT (G) PER SERVING	SATURATED FAT (G) PER SERVING	TRANS FAT (G) PER SERVING	SAT + TRANS (G)
	Caesar Salad (without chicken)	7.5 oz (213 g)	90	4	2.5	0	2.5
	California Cobb Salad with Grilled Chicken	11.7 oz (334 g)	280	11	5	0	5
	California Cobb Salad with Crispy Chicken	11.9 oz (338 g)	360	18	6	1.5	7.5
	California Cobb Salad (without chicken)	8.4 oz (237 g)	160	9	4	0	4
	Fruit & Walnut Salad	9.3 oz (264 g)	310	13	2	0	2
	Side Salad	3.1 oz (87 g)	20	0	0	0	0
	Butter Garlic Croutons	0.5 oz (14 g)	60	1	0	0	0
Desserts and Shakes	Fruit 'n Yogurt Parfait	5.3 oz (149 g)	160	2	1	0	1
	Fruit 'n Yogurt Parfait (without granola)	5 oz (142 g)	130	2	1	0	1
	Apple Dippers with Low Fat Caramel Dip	3.2 oz (89 g)	100	1	0.5	0	0.5
	Apple Dippers	1 pkg (68 g)	35	0	0	0	0
	Low Fat Caramel Dip	0.8 oz (21 g)	70	0.5	0	0	0
	Vanilla Reduced Fat Ice Cream Cone	3.2 oz (90 g)	150	3.5	2	0	2
	Kiddie Cone	1 oz (29 g)	45	1	0.5	0	0.5
	Strawberry Sundae	6.3 oz (178 g)	280	6	3.5	0	3.5
	Hot Caramel Sundae	6.4 oz (182 g)	340	7	4.5	0	4.5
	Hot Fudge Sundae	6.3 oz (179 g)	330	9	6	0	6
	Peanuts (for Sundaes)	0.3 oz (7 g)	45	3.5	0.5	0	0.5
	McFlurry with M&M's Candies (12 fl oz cup)	12.3 oz (348 g)	620	20	12	1	13
	McFlurry with Oreo Cookies (12 fl oz cup)	11.9 oz (337 g)	560	16	9	2	11
	Chocolate Triple Thick Shake (12 fl oz cup)	333 ml	440	10	6	0.5	6.5
	Chocolate Triple Thick Shake (16 fl oz cup)	444 ml	580	14	8	1	9
	Chocolate Triple Thick Shake (21 fl oz cup)	583 ml	770	18	11	1	12
	Chocolate Triple Thick Shake (32 fl oz cup)	888 ml	1160	27	16	2	18

Item	Serving					
Strawberry Triple Thick Shake (12 fl oz cup)	333 ml	420	10	6	0.5	6.5
Strawberry Triple Thick Shake (16 fl oz cup)	444 ml	560	13	8	1	9
Strawberry Triple Thick Shake (21 fl oz cup)	583 ml	740	18	11	1	12
Strawberry Triple Thick Shake (32 fl oz cup)	888 ml	1110	26	16	2	18
Vanilla Triple Thick Shake (12 fl oz cup)	333 ml	420	10	6	0.5	6.5
Vanilla Triple Thick Shake (16 fl oz cup)	444 ml	550	13	8	1	9
Vanilla Triple Thick Shake (21 fl oz cup)	583 ml	740	18	11	1	12
Vanilla Triple Thick Shake (32 fl oz cup)	888 ml	1110	26	16	2	18
Baked Apple Pie	77 g	250	11	3	4.5	7.5
McDonaldland Chocolate Chip Cookies	56 g	270	11	6	0	6
McDonaldland Cookies	57 g	250	8	2	2.5	4.5
Chocolate Chip Cookie	1 cookie	160	7	2	1.5	3.5
Oatmeal Raisin Cookie	1 cookie	140	5	1	1	2
Sugar Cookie	1 cookie	150	6	1	1.5	2.5

PIZZA HUT

Pizza

Item	Serving					
Individual Chicken Supreme 4forAll Pizzas	274 g	580	23	9	3	12
Individual Meat Lover's 4forAll Pizzas	283 g	760	41	17	3.5	20.5
Individual Pepperoni Lover's 4forAll Pizzas	269 g	760	41	18	3.5	21.5
Individual Sausage Lover's 4forAll Pizzas	266 g	720	38	15	3.5	18.5
Individual Super Supreme 4forAll Pizzas	315 g	750	39	16	3.5	19.5
Individual Supreme 4forAll Pizzas	290 g	710	36	15	3.5	18.5
Individual Veggie Lover's 4forAll Pizzas	258 g	550	23	9	3	12
Individual Meat Lover's Pan Pizza 6" Personal Pan Pizza	301 g	800	41	16	1	17
Individual Pan Pizza 6" Personal Pan Pizza	250 g	630	27	12	1	13

BRAND NAME	PRODUCT NAME	SERVING SIZE	CALORIES PER SERVING	TOTAL FAT (G) PER SERVING	SATURATED FAT (G) PER SERVING	TRANS FAT (G) PER SERVING	SAT + TRANS (G)
	Individual Pepperoni Lover's Pan Pizza 6" Personal Pan Pizza	1 pizza	800	42	17	1	18
	Individual Sausage Lover's Pan Pizza 6" Personal Pan Pizza	1 pizza	750	38	15	1	16
	Individual Veggie Lover's Pan Pizza 6" Personal Pan Pizza	1 pizza	580	23	9	0.5	9.5
	Stuffed Crust	1 slice	370	14	8	1	9
	Thin 'N Crispy Pizza 12" Medium	1 slice	200	8	4.5	0	4.5
	P'Zone Classic	½ pizza	610	21	11	0	11
	Fit 'N Delicious 12" Medium Chicken & Veggie	1 pizza	160	4.5	2	0	2
	Fit 'N Delicious 12" Medium Ham & Veggie	1 pizza	150	4	2	0	2
	Fit 'N Delicious 12" Medium Veggie	1 pizza	140	4	1.5	0	1.5
Appetizers	Bread Stick	1	270	8	1.5	0	1.5
	Cheese Bread Stick	1	320	11	3.5	0	3.5
	Cheese Garlic Bread	1 piece	240	17	6	0	6
	Garlic Bread	1 piece	170	12	2.5	0	2.5
	Chicken Munchers	2	80	3.5	0.5	0	0.5
	Hot Wings	2	110	6	2	0	2
	Jalapeño Poppers	2	140	8	3.5	0	3.5
	Mild Wings	2	110	7	2	0	2
	Mozzarella Sticks	2	150	8	3.5	0	3.5
	Onion Rings	2.5 oz.	180	9	1.5	0	1.5
	FreshExpress—Ranch Salad Kit	100 g	110	8	0.5	0	0.5

Pasta

Item	Serving	Cal				
Cavatini	416 g	420	15	7	0	7
Cavatini Supreme	452 g	460	18	8	0	8
Pasta Bakes Marinara	510 g	840	32	4.5	0	4.5
Pasta Bakes Marinara with Meatballs	567 g	1050	42	10	0	10
Pasta Bakes Primavera	540 g	970	43	10	0	10
Pasta Bakes Primavera with Chicken	540 g	1050	50	12	0	12
Spaghetti with Marinara Sauce	639 g	490	8	1.5	0	1.5
Spaghetti with Meat Sauce	696 g	640	20	7	0	7
Spaghetti with Meatballs	696 g	630	19	7	0	7

Dessert

Item	Serving	Cal				
Apple Dessert Pizza	1 slice	260	3.5	0.5	0	0.5
Cherry Dessert Pizza	1 slice	240	3.5	0.5	0	0.5
White Icing Dipping Cup	2 oz.	190	0	0	0	0
Cinnamon Sticks	2 pieces	170	5	1	0	1

TACO BELL

Gorditas

Item	Serving	Cal				
Regular Style Gordita Baja—Beef	153 g	350	19	5	0.5	5.5
Regular Style Gordita Baja—Chicken	153 g	320	15	3.5	0	3.5
Regular Style Gordita Baja—Steak	153 g	320	16	4	0	4
Regular Style Gordita Supreme—Chicken	153 g	290	12	5	0	5
Regular Style Gordita Supreme—Steak	153 g	290	13	6	0.5	6.5
Regular Style Gordita Supreme—Beef	153 g	300	13	4	1.5	5.5
Regular Style Gordita Nacho Cheese—Chicken	153 g	270	10	2.5	1	3.5
Regular Style Gordita Nacho Cheese—Steak	153 g	270	11	3	1.5	4.5

BRAND NAME	PRODUCT NAME	SERVING SIZE	CALORIES PER SERVING	TOTAL FAT (G) PER SERVING	SATURATED FAT (G) PER SERVING	TRANS FAT (G) PER SERVING	SAT + TRANS (G)
Chalupas	Regular Style Chalupa Baja—Beef	153 g	430	28	7	2	9
	Regular Style Chalupa Baja—Chicken	153 g	400	24	5	2	7
	Regular Style Chalupa Baja—Steak	153 g	410	25	6	2	8
	Regular Style Chalupa Nacho Cheese—Beef	153 g	380	22	5	3	8
	Regular Style Chalupa Nacho Cheese—Chicken	153 g	350	18	4	3	7
	Regular Style Chalupa Nacho Cheese—Steak	153 g	360	20	4.5	3	7.5
	Regular Style Chalupa Supreme—Beef	153 g	400	24	8	2.5	10.5
	Regular Style Chalupa Supreme—Chicken	153 g	370	21	7	2	9
	Regular Style Chalupa Supreme—Steak	153 g	370	22	7	2	9
Tacos	Fresco Style Chicken Ranchero Taco	113 g	170	4	1	0.5	1.5
	Fresco Style Grilled Steak Soft Taco	128 g	170	5	1.5	0.5	2
	Fresco Style Soft Taco—Beef	113 g	190	8	2.5	1	3.5
	Fresco Style Soft Taco Supreme—Beef	128 g	190	8	2.5	1	3.5
	Fresco Style Taco	92 g	150	7	2.5	0.5	3
	Fresco Style Taco Supreme	106 g	150	7	2.5	0.5	3
	Regular Style Chicken Ranchero Taco	135 g	270	14	4	0.5	4.5
	Regular Style Grilled Steak Soft Taco	128 g	280	17	4.5	1	5.5
	Regular Style Soft Taco—Beef	99 g	210	10	4	1	5
	Regular Style Soft Taco Supreme—Beef	135 g	260	14	7	1	8
	Regular Style Taco	78 g	170	10	4	0.5	4.5
	Regular Style Taco Supreme	113 g	220	14	7	1	8
Specialties	Fresco Style Enchirito—Beef	206 g	270	9	3	1	4
	Fresco Style Enchirito—Chicken	206 g	250	5	1.5	1	2.5

	Weight (g)	Calories				
Fresco Style Enchirito—Steak	206 g	250	7	2	1	3
Fresco Style Express Taco Salad with Chips	464 g	510	23	7	3	10
Fresco Style Fiesta Taco Salad	534 g	760	37	9	5	14
Fresco Style Mexican Pizza	209 g	450	23	5	3	8
Fresco Style MexiMelt	120 g	190	8	2.5	1	3.5
Fresco Style Southwest Steak Bowl	436 g	570	17	4	2.5	6.5
Fresco Style Tostada	177 g	200	6	1	1	2
Fresco Style Zesty Chicken Border Bowl	411 g	470	14	2.5	2.5	5
Regular Style Cheese Quesadilla	142 g	490	28	13	2	15
Regular Style Chicken Quesadilla	184 g	540	30	13	2	15
Regular Style Enchirito—Beef	213 g	380	18	9	1.5	10.5
Regular Style Enchirito—Chicken	213 g	350	14	7	1.5	8.5
Regular Style Enchirito—Steak	213 g	360	16	8	1.5	9.5
Regular Style Express Taco Salad with Chips	479 g	600	32	12	3.5	15.5
Regular Style Fiesta Taco Salad	548 g	860	46	14	5	19
Regular Style Mexican Pizza	216 g	540	31	10	3.5	13.5
Regular Style MexiMelt	128 g	290	16	8	1	9
Regular Style Southwest Steak Bowl	443 g	690	28	8	2.5	10.5
Regular Style Steak Quesadilla	184 g	540	31	14	2	16
Regular Style Tostada	170 g	250	10	4	1.5	5.5
Regular Style Zesty Chicken Border Bowl	418 g	730	40	8	2.5	10.5

Nachos and Sides

	Weight (g)	Calories				
Fresco Style Mexican Rice	138 g	150	4	0.5	0.5	1
Fresco Style Nachos	64 g	200	11	2	2	4
Fresco Style Nachos BellGrande	252 g	590	29	6	5	11
Fresco Style Nachos Supreme	167 g	340	17	4.5	2.5	7
Fresco Style Pintos 'n Cheese	135 g	130	2.5	0.5	1	1.5
Regular Style Cinnamon Twists	35 g	160	5	1	1	2

BRAND NAME	PRODUCT NAME	SERVING SIZE	CALORIES PER SERVING	TOTAL FAT (G) PER SERVING	SATURATED FAT (G) PER SERVING	TRANS FAT (G) PER SERVING	SAT + TRANS (G)
	Regular Style Mexican Rice	131 g	200	9	3.5	0.5	4
	Regular Style Nachos	99 g	300	18	4	4	8
	Regular Style Nachos BellGrande	308 g	730	41	12	7	19
	Regular Style Nachos Supreme	195 g	430	25	8	3.5	11.5
	Regular Style Pintos 'n Cheese	128 g	180	7	3.5	1	2.5
WENDY'S Sandwiches	Jr. Hamburger	117 g	280	9	3.5	0.5	4
	Jr. Cheeseburger	129 g	320	13	6	0.5	6.5
	Jr. Cheeseburger Deluxe	179 g	360	16	6	0.5	6.5
	Jr. Bacon Cheeseburger	165 g	380	18	7	0.5	7.5
	Hamburger, Kid's Meal	110 g	270	9	3.5	0.5	4
	Cheeseburger, Kid's Meal	120 g	320	13	6	0.5	6.5
	Classic Single with Everything	218 g	420	19	7	1	8
	Big Bacon Classic	282 g	580	29	12	1.5	13.5
	Ultimate Chicken Grill Sandwich	225 g	360	7	1.5	0	1.5
	Spicy Chicken Fillet Sandwich	224 g	510	18	3.5	1.5	5
	Homestyle Chicken Fillet Sandwich	230 g	540	22	4	1.5	5.5
Side Selections	Side Salad	166 g	35	0	0	0	0
	Cesear Side Salad	99 g	70	4.5	2	0	2
	Mandarin Orange Cup	142 g	80	0	0	0	0
	Low Fat Strawberry Yogurt and Granola Topping	215 g	310	6.5	1.5	0	1.5
	Plain Baked Potato	283 g	270	0	0	0	0
	Sour Cream & Chives Baked Potato	311 g	320	4	2	0	2

Item	Serving					
Broccoli & Cheese Baked Potato	397 g	340	3.5	1	0	1
Bacon & Cheese Baked Potato	366 g	460	13	5	0	5
Chili (small)	227 g	220	6	2.5	0	2.5
French Fries (medium)	142 g	440	21	3.5	5	8.5
Homestyle Chicken Strips and Crispy Chicken Nuggets						
Homestyle Chicken Strips	159 g	410	18	3.5	3	6.5
5 Piece Nugget	75 g	220	14	3	1.5	4.5
Garden Sensations Salads and Fresh Fruit						
Mandarin Chicken Salad	348 g	170	2	0.5	0	0.5
Spring Mix Salad	313 g	180	11	6	0	6
Chicken BLT Salad	374 g	340	18	9	0	9
Taco Supremo Salad	494 g	380	17	9	0.5	9.5
Homestyle Chicken Strips Salad	417 g	450	22	8	2.5	10.5
Desserts						
Frosty (medium)	298 g	430	11	7	0	7
JACK IN THE BOX						
Breakfast						
Bacon, Egg & Cheese Biscuit	149 g	430	25	8	5	13
Blueberry French Toast Sticks	121 g	450	20	4.5	4.5	9
Breakfast Jack	125 g	290	12	4.5	0	4.5
Chicken Biscuit	154 g	450	24	6	6	12
Ciabatta Breakfast Sandwich	284 g	740	38	10	1	11
Extreme Sausage Sandwich	213 g	670	48	17	1.5	18.5
Hash Brown	57 g	150	10	2.5	3	5.5
Meaty Breakfast Burrito	183 g	480	29	10	1	11
Original French Toast Sticks	121 g	470	23	5	5	10
Sausage Biscuit	131 g	440	29	8	5	13
Sausage Breakfast Jack	154 g	450	28	10	1	11
Sausage Croissant	174 g	580	39	13	4	17

BRAND NAME	PRODUCT NAME	SERVING SIZE	CALORIES PER SERVING	TOTAL FAT (G) PER SERVING	SATURATED FAT (G) PER SERVING	TRANS FAT (G) PER SERVING	SAT + TRANS (G)
	Sausage, Egg & Cheese Biscuit	234 g	740	55	17	6	23
	Sourdough Breakfast Sandwich	156 g	420	24	8	2	10
	Spicy Chicken Biscuit	169 g	460	22	5	7	12
	Supreme Croissant	151 g	450	25	9	3.5	12.5
	Ultimate Breakfast Sandwich	249 g	570	27	10	1	11
Salads (no dressing)	Asian Chicken Salad	401 g	140	1	0	0	0
	Chicken Caesar Salad	336 g	220	8	4	0	4
	Chicken Club Salad	431 g	300	15	6	0	6
	Side Salad	137 g	60	3	1.5	0	1.5
	Southwest Chicken Salad	488 g	330	13	6	0	6
Burgers	Bacon Bacon Cheeseburger	294 g	840	56	19	1.5	20.5
	Bacon Ultimate Cheeseburger	338 g	1090	77	30	3	33
	Bacon 'n' Cheese Ciabatta Burger	395 g	1140	79	28	3	31
	Hamburger	118 g	310	14	6	1	7
	Hamburger with Cheese	131 g	350	17	8	1	9
	Hamburger Deluxe	169 g	370	21	7	1	8
	Hamburger Deluxe with Cheese	194 g	460	28	11	1	12
	Jumbo Jack	261 g	600	35	12	1.5	13.5
	Jumbo Jack with Cheese	286 g	690	42	16	1.5	17.5
	Junior Bacon Cheeseburger	131 g	430	25	9	1	10
	Original Ciabatta Burger	307 g	720	42	13	1.5	14.5
	Sourdough Jack	245 g	710	51	18	3	21
	Sourdough Ultimate Cheeseburger	291 g	950	73	29	4.5	33.5
	Ultimate Cheeseburger	323 g	1010	71	28	3	33

Chicken and More	Bacon Chicken Sandwich	152 g	440	24	6	2.5	8.5
	Bruschetta Chicken Ciabatta Sandwich	338 g	660	26	7	0	7
	Chicken Breast Strips	201 g	500	25	6	6	12
	Chicken Fajita Pita	218 g	300	10	4.5	0	4.5
	Chicken Sandwich	145 g	400	21	4.5	2.5	7
	Classic Chicken Ciabatta Sandwich	300 g	510	13	2.5	0	2.5
	Fish & Chips	252 g	680	41	10	14	24
	Jack's Spicy Chicken	270 g	620	31	6	3	9
	Jack's Spicy Chicken with Cheese	294 g	700	37	10	3	13
	Sourdough Grilled Chicken Club	266 g	530	28	7	2	9
	Southwest Pita	179 g	260	4.5	1	0	1
	Ultimate Club Sandwich	277 g	570	32	10	2	12
Snacks and Extras	Bacon Cheddar Potato Wedges	217 g	560	36	12	6	18
	Egg Roll	1	130	6	2	1	3
	Egg Rolls	3	400	19	6	3	9
	Monster Beef Taco	112 g	240	14	5	2	7
	Natural Cut Fries, small	99 g	270	12	3	3.5	6.5
	Natural Cut Fries, medium	133 g	360	17	4	5	9
	Natural Cut Fries, large	196 g	530	25	6	7	12
	Onion Rings	119 g	500	30	6	10	16
	Regular Beef Taco	76 g	160	8	3	1	4
	Seasoned Curly Fries, small	84 g	270	15	3	5	8
	Seasoned Curly Fries, medium	125 g	400	23	5	7	12
	Seasoned Curly Fries, large	170 g	550	31	6	10	16
	Stuffed Jalapenos	3	230	13	6	2	8
	Stuffed Jalapenos	7	530	30	13	4.5	17.5

BRAND NAME	PRODUCT NAME	SERVING SIZE	CALORIES PER SERVING	TOTAL FAT (G) PER SERVING	SATURATED FAT (G) PER SERVING	TRANS FAT (G) PER SERVING	SAT + TRANS (G)
Shakes and Desserts	Cheesecake	103 g	310	16	9	1	10
	Chocolate Ice Cream Shake, small	315 g	660	29	18	1	19
	Chocolate Ice Cream Shake, medium	413 g	850	38	24	1.5	25.5
	Chocolate Ice Cream Shake, large	630 g	1310	57	36	2	38
	Chocolate Malted Crunch Ice Cream Shake, small	329 g	720	33	22	1	23
	Chocolate Malted Crunch Ice Cream Shake, medium	427 g	920	43	28	1.5	19.5
	Chocolate Malted Crunch Ice Cream Shake, large	659 g	1450	65	43	2.5	45.5
	Double Fudge Cake	85 g	310	11	3	0.5	3.5
	Oreo Cookie Ice Cream Shake, small	301 g	670	33	19	3	22
	Oreo Cookie Ice Cream Shake, medium	399 g	870	43	25	3.5	28.5
	Oreo Cookie Ice Cream Shake, large	601 g	1350	66	37	6	43
	Strawberry Banana Ice Cream Shake, small	344 g	700	28	18	1	19
	Strawberry Banana Ice Cream Shake, medium	442 g	900	38	24	1.5	25.5
	Strawberry Banana Ice Cream Shake, large	688 g	1410	56	35	2	37
	Strawberry Ice Cream Shake, small	313 g	640	28	18	1	19
	Strawberry Ice Cream Shake, medium	411 g	830	38	24	1.5	25.5
	Strawberry Ice Cream Shake, large	626 g	1270	56	35	2	37
	Vanilla Ice Cream Shake, small	285 g	570	29	18	1	19
	Vanilla Ice Cream Shake, medium	373 g	750	38	24	1.5	25.5
	Vanilla Ice Cream Shake, large	570 g	1140	58	36	2.5	38.5
Kids' Meals	Applesauce (1 cup)	113 g	100	0	0	0	0
	Chicken Breast Strips	100 g	250	12	3	3	6
	Hamburger	118 g	310	14	6	1	7
	Hamburger with cheese	131 g	350	17	8	1	9
	Natural Cut Fries, kid's portion	79 g	210	10	2.5	3	5.5

DAIRY QUEEN

Breakfast

	Serving	Calories	Total Fat (g)	Saturated Fat (g)	Trans Fat (g)	Sat + Trans Fat (g)
Biscuit	62 g	230	12	3	3	6
Sausage patty	33 g	110	9	3.5	0	3.5
Bacon	2 strips	80	7	3	0	3
Ham	1 slice	40	1.5	0.5	0	0.5
Biscuits & Gravy	295 g	780	35	10	8	18
Buttermilk Pancakes with syrup & 1 butter packet	198 g	530	22	3	5	8
Cinnamon Roll with glaze	170 g	630	26	6	7	13
Hashbrown Patty	62 g	160	11	2.5	2.5	5
Ultimate Hashbrowns Platter with sausage	431 g	810	55	20	6	26
Ultimate Hashbrowns Platter with ham	422 g	650	40	14	4	18
Ultimate Hashbrowns Platter with bacon	384 g	700	47	16	6	22
Sausage & Egg Biscuit (no cheese)	152 g	400	24	8	3	11
Ham & Egg Biscuit (no cheese)	147 g	320	17	5	3	8
Bacon & Egg Biscuit (no cheese)	131 g	360	21	6	3	9
American Cheese	1 slice	50	4.5	2.5	0	2.5

GrillBurgers

	Serving	Calories				
Classic GrillBurger, no cheese	240 g	600	33	12	3	15
½ lb GrillBurger, no cheese	326 g	860	53	21	5	26
Bacon Cheese GrillBurger	247 g	750	46	19	4	23
Mushroom Swiss GrillBurger	221 g	750	49	16	4	20
California GrillBurger	219 g	690	44	13	4	17

Hot Sandwiches

	Serving	Calories				
Grilled Turkey Sandwich	281 g	730	45	10	5	15
Grilled Chicken Sandwich	217 g	520	26	4.5	2	6.5
Crispy Chicken Sandwich	240 g	690	37	6	4	10

Hot Dogs

	Serving	Calories				
Classic Hot Dog	148 g	400	27	11	1.5	12.5
Classic Chili Cheese Dog	205 g	510	35	15	2	17

BRAND NAME	PRODUCT NAME	SERVING SIZE	CALORIES PER SERVING	TOTAL FAT (G) PER SERVING	SATURATED FAT (G) PER SERVING	TRANS FAT (G) PER SERVING	SAT + TRANS (G)
Salads	House Salad Entree	316 g	120	5	3	0	3
	Crispy Chicken Salad	392 g	350	20	6	2.5	8.5
	Grilled Chicken Salad	389 g	240	10	5	0	5
	Crispy Chicken Caesar Salad	215 g	280	16	5	2.5	7.5
	Grilled Chicken Caesar Salad	213 g	170	7	3	0	3
	Side Salad, no dressing	126 g	60	2.5	1.5	0	1.5
	DQ Honey Mustard Dressing	57 g	260	21	3.5	0	3.5
	Wish-Bone Fat Free Italian Dressing	43 g	25	0	0	0	0
	DQ Bleu Cheese Dressing	57 g	210	20	4	0	4
	DQ Caesar Dressing	57 g	330	34	6	0.5	6.5
	DQ Ranch Dressing	57 g	310	33	5	0.5	5.5
Entrees	Chicken Strips	4	400	24	4.5	5	9.5
	Chicken Strips	6	600	35	7	7	14
	Buffalo Chicken Strips	4	540	30	6	6	12
	Buffalo Chicken Strips	6	810	45	9	8	17
	Fish Fillets, no tartar sauce	4	440	24	8	5	13
	Fish Fillets, no tartar sauce	6	660	36	12	8	16
	Tartar Sauce	2 oz.	220	24	3	0	3
	Chicken Quesadilla	212 g	550	31	17	2	19
	Vegetable Quesadilla	156 g	440	25	13	2	15
French Fries, Sides and Appetizers	French Fries	5 oz.	380	15	3	4	7
	French Fries	7 oz.	530	21	4	6	10
	Onion Rings	4 oz.	470	30	6	7	13
	Onion Rings	5 oz.	590	37	7	9	16

Blizzard Flavor Treats						
Small Oreo Cookies Blizzard	283 g	570	21	10	2.5	12.5
Medium Oreo Cookies Blizzard	334 g	700	26	12	4	14
Large Oreo Cookies Blizzard	500 g	1010	37	18	5	23
Small Choc. Chip Cook. Dough Blizzard	319 g	720	28	14	2.5	16.5
Medium Choc. Chip Cook. Dough Blizzard	446 g	1030	40	20	4	24
Large Choc. Chip Cook. Dough Blizzard	560 g	1320	52	26	5	31
Small Banana Split Blizzard	297 g	460	14	9	0	9
Medium Banana Split Blizzard	382 g	580	17	11	0.5	11.5
Large Banana Split Blizzard	527 g	810	23	15	1	16
Cones						
Small Vanilla Cone	142 g	230	7	4.5	0	4.5
Medium Vanilla Cone	198 g	330	9	6	0	6
Large Vanilla Cone	284 g	480	15	9	0.5	9.5
Small Dipped Cone	156 g	340	17	9	1	10
Medium Dipped Cone	220 g	490	24	13	1.5	14.5
Large Dipped Cone	312 g	710	36	17	2.5	19.5
Royal Treats						
Classic Banana Split	369 g	510	12	8	0	8
Peanut Butter Blast	269 g	700	37	19	0	19
Peanut Butter Parfait	305 g	730	31	17	0	17
Brownie Earthquake	304 g	740	27	16	3	19
Strawberry Shortcake	241 g	430	14	9	1	10
Pecan Praline Parfait	305 g	720	29	11	0.5	11.5
Novelties						
Starkiss Bar	85 g	80	0	0	0	0
DQ Fudge Bar	66 g	50	0	0	0	0
DQ Vanilla Orange Bar	66 g	60	0	0	0	0
Chocolate Dilly Bar	85 g	210	13	7	0	7
Buster Bar	149 g	450	28	12	1	13

BRAND NAME	PRODUCT NAME	SERVING SIZE	CALORIES PER SERVING	TOTAL FAT (G) PER SERVING	SATURATED FAT (G) PER SERVING	TRANS FAT (G) PER SERVING	SAT + TRANS (G)
Curly Shakes and Malts	Small Chocolate Curly Shake	411 g	620	18	11	0.5	11.5
	Medium Chocolate Curly Shake	539 g	820	23	15	0.5	15.5
	Large Chocolate Curly Shake	794 g	1200	34	22	1	23
	Small Strawberry Curly Shake	411 g	540	17	11	0.5	11.5
	Medium Strawberry Curly Shake	539 g	710	22	14	0.5	14.5
	Large Strawberry Curly Shake	794 g	1040	33	21	1	22
Sundaes	Small Chocolate Sundae	163 g	280	7	4.5	0	4.5
	Medium Chocolate Sundae	234 g	400	10	6	0	6
	Large Chocolate Sundae	333 g	580	15	10	0	10
	Small Strawberry Sundae	163 g	240	7	4.5	0	4.5
	Medium Strawberry Sundae	234 g	340	9	6	0	6
	Large Strawberry Sundae	333 g	500	15	9	0	9
Misty	Small Cherry Misty	442 g	210	0	0	0	0
	Medium Cherry Misty	580 g	280	0	0	0	0
	Large Cherry Misty	884 g	430	0	0	0	0
	Small Grape Misty	442 g	240	0	0	0	0
	Medium Grape Misty	580 g	320	0	0	0	0
	Large Grape Misty	884 g	480	0	0	0	0
	Small Lemon Lime Misty	442 g	140	0	0	0	0
	Medium Lemon Lime Misty	580 g	190	0	0	0	0
	Large Lemon Lime Misty	884 g	280	0	0	0	0

	Weight	Calories				
Breakfast Sandwiches on Deli Round						
Cheese	135 g	270	9	4	0	4
Chipotle Steak & Cheese	213 g	470	25	9	0.5	9.5
Double Bacon & Cheese	179 g	460	23	12	0.5	12.5
Honey Mustard Ham & Egg	171 g	270	5	1.5	0	1.5
Western with Cheese	190 g	360	14	7	0	7
Breakfast Sandwiches on 6-inch Bread						
Cheese	156 g	310	9	3.5	0	3.5
Chipotle Steak & Cheese	234 g	510	25	9	0.5	9.5
Double Bacon & Cheese	200 g	500	23	12	0.5	12.5
Honey Mustard Ham & Egg	192 g	310	5	1.5	0	1.5
Western with Cheese	211 g	400	14	7	0	7
Breakfast Wraps						
Cheese	148 g	220	10	3.5	0	3.5
Chipotle Steak & Cheese	226 g	430	27	8	0	8
Double Bacon & Cheese	192 g	420	25	11	0.5	11.5
Honey Mustard Ham & Egg	184 g	230	7	1	0	1
Western with Cheese	203 g	310	16	6	0	6
6-inch Sandwiches (with 6 grams of fat or less; includes Italian bread, lettuce, tomatoes, onions, green peppers, pickles, and olives)						
Ham	224 g	290	5	1.5	0	1.5
Oven Roasted Chicken Breast	238 g	330	5	1.5	0	1.5
Roast Beef	224 g	290	5	2	0	2
Turkey Breast	224 g	280	4.5	1.5	0	1.5
Turkey Breast & Ham	234 g	290	5	1.5	0	1.5
Subway Club	257 g	320	6	2	0	2
Sweet Onion Chicken Teriyaki	281 g	370	5	1.5	0	1.5
Veggie Delite	167 g	230	3	1	0	1

BRAND NAME	PRODUCT NAME	SERVING SIZE	CALORIES PER SERVING	TOTAL FAT (G) PER SERVING	SATURATED FAT (G) PER SERVING	TRANS FAT (G) PER SERVING	SAT + TRANS (G)
6-inch Sandwiches (includes Italian bread, lettuce, tomatoes, onions, green peppers, pickles, and olives)	Cheese Steak	250 g	360	10	4.5	0	4.5
	Chicken & Bacon Ranch	297 g	530	25	10	0.5	10.5
	Chicken Parmesan	315 g	510	18	6	0	6
	Chipotle Southwest Cheese Steak	271 g	450	20	6	0	6
	Tuna	250 g	530	31	7	0.5	7.5
	Cold Cut Combo	249 g	410	17	7	0.5	7.5
	Italian BMT	243 g	450	21	8	0	8
	Meatball Marinara	377 g	560	24	11	1	12
	Spicy Italian	227 g	480	25	9	0	9
	Subway Melt	254 g	382	12	5	0	5
Deli-Style Sandwiches (includes deli roll, lettuce, tomatoes, onions, green peppers, pickles, and olives)	Tuna with cheese	161 g	350	18	5	0.5	5.5
	Ham	142 g	210	4	1.5	0	1.5
	Roast Beef	152 g	220	4.5	2	0	2
	Turkey Breast	152 g	210	3.5	1.5	0	1.5
Wraps	Chicken & Bacon Ranch with cheese	257 g	440	27	10	0.5	10.5
	Tuna with cheese	209 g	440	32	6	0.5	6.5
	Turkey Breast & Bacon Melt with chipotle sauce	228 g	380	24	7	0	7
	Turkey Breast	184 g	190	6	1	0	1
Salads (dressing and croutons not included)	Grilled Chicken & Baby Spinach	300 g	140	3	1	0	1
	Subway Club	412 g	160	4	1.5	0	1.5
	Tuna with cheese	404 g	360	29	6	0.5	6.5
	Veggie Delite	322 g	60	1	0	0	0

	Serving	Calories				
Salad Dressing						
Atkins Honey Mustard	57 g	200	22	3	0	3
Fat Free Italian	57 g	35	0	0	0	0
Ranch	57 g	200	22	3.5	0	3.5
6-inch Double Meat						
DM Turkey Breast	281 g	340	6	1.5	0	1.5
DM Turkey Breast & Ham	300 g	360	7	2	0	2
DM Ham	302 g	380	7	2.5	0	2.5
DM Roast Beef	281 g	360	7	3.5	0	3.5
DM Subway Club	347 g	420	8	3.5	0	3.5
DM Oven Roasted Chicken	309 g	430	8	2	0	2
DM Classic Tuna	320 g	790	55	11	1	12
DM Seafood Sensation	320 g	640	38	8	1	9
DM Italian BMT	306 g	630	35	14	0	14
DM Cold Cut Combo	320 g	550	28	10	1	11
DM Turkey Breast, Ham & Bacon Melt	330 g	500	17	8	0	8
DM Cheese Steak	320 g	450	14	6	0	6
DM Meatball Marinara	575 g	960	42	18	2	20
DM Sweet Onion Chicken Teriyaki	373 g	490	7	2	0	2
DM Chipotle Southwest Cheese Steak	342 g	540	24	7	0	7
Soup (10-oz. cup)						
Brown and Wild Rice with Chicken	310 g	230	11	3.5	0	3.5
Chicken and Dumpling	310 g	140	3.5	1.5	0	1.5
Chili Con Carne	310 g	340	11	5	0	5
Cream of Broccoli	310 g	140	5	2	0	2
Cream of Potato with Bacon	310 g	220	10	4	0	4
Golden Broccoli & Cheese	310 g	180	11	5	0	5
Minestrone	310 g	90	1	0	0	0
New England Style Clam Chowder	310 g	150	5	1.5	0	1.5

BRAND NAME	PRODUCT NAME	SERVING SIZE	CALORIES PER SERVING	TOTAL FAT (G) PER SERVING	SATURATED FAT (G) PER SERVING	TRANS FAT (G) PER SERVING	SAT + TRANS (G)
	Roasted Chicken Noodle	310 g	90	2	0.5	0	0.5
	Spanish Style Chicken with Rice	310 g	110	2.5	1	0	1
	Tomato Garden Vegetable with Rotini	310 g	90	0.5	0	0	0
	Vegetable Beef	310 g	100	1.5	0.5	0	0.5
Breads	6-inch Italian (White) Bread	71 g	190	2.5	1.5	0	1.5
	6-inch Wheat Bread	78 g	200	2.5	1	0	1
	6-inch Parmesan Oregano Bread	75 g	210	3.5	1.5	0.5	2
	6-inch Honey Oat	88 g	250	3.5	1	0	1
	6-inch Hearty Italian Bread	75 g	210	2.5	1.5	0	1.5
	6-inch Monterey Cheddar	82 g	240	6	3.5	0.5	4
	6-inch Italian Herbs & Cheese	82 g	240	6	3	1	4
	Deli-Style Roll	71 g	170	2.5	1	0	1
	Carb Conscious Wrap	70 g	120	4.5	0.5	0	0.5
Sandwich Condiments (amount on 6-inch sub)	Bacon	2 strips	45	3.5	1.5	0	1.5
	Chipotle Southwest Sauce	21 g	100	10	1.5	0	1.5
	Honey Mustard Sauce	21 g	30	0	0	0	0
	Light Mayonnaise	15 g	50	5	1	0	1
	Mayonnaise	15 g	110	12	2	0	2
	Mustard (yellow or deli brown)	2 tsp	5	0	0	0	0
	Olive Oil Blend	1 tsp	45	5	0	0	0
	Ranch Dressing	21 g	70	8	1	0	1
	Red Wine Vinaigrette, Fat Free	21 g	30	0	0	0	0
	Sweet Onion Sauce, Fat Free	21 g	40	0	0	0	0
	Vinegar	1 tsp	0	0	0	0	0

Cheese (amount on 6-inch sub, wrap, or salad)

American	11 g	40	3.5	2	0	2
Monterey Cheddar, shredded	14 g	50	4.5	3	0	3
Natural Cheddar	15 g	60	5	3	0	3
Pepperjack	14 g	50	4	2.5	0	2.5
Provolone	14 g	50	4	2	0	2
Swiss	14 g	50	4.5	2.5	0	2.5

Cookies

Chocolate Chip	45 g	210	10	4	1	5
Chocolate Chunk	45 g	220	10	3.5	2.5	6
Double Chocolate Chip	45 g	210	10	4	1	5
M&M	45 g	210	10	3.5	2.5	6
Oatmeal Raisin	45 g	200	8	2.5	2.5	5
Peanut Butter	45 g	220	12	4	1	5
Sugar	45 g	230	12	3.5	3.5	7
White Chip Macadamia Nut	45 g	220	11	3.5	1	4.5

HARDEE'S

Breakfast

Loaded Breakfast Burrito	258 g	780	51	20	n/l	n/a
Made-from-Scratch Biscuit	109 g	370	23	5	n/l	n/a
Egg Biscuit	152 g	450	29	6	n/l	n/a
Bacon Biscuit	120 g	430	28	7	n/l	n/a
Sausage Biscuit	142 g	530	38	10	n/l	n/a
Country Ham Biscuit	144 g	440	26	6	n/l	n/a
Chicken Fillet Biscuit	226 g	600	34	7	n/l	n/a
Country Steak Biscuit	180 g	620	41	11	n/l	n/a
Breaded Pork Chop Biscuit	222 g	690	42	8	n/l	n/a
Grilled Pork Chop Biscuit	208 g	560	35	9	n/l	n/a
Sausage & Egg Biscuit	185 g	610	44	11	n/l	n/a
Country Steak & Egg Biscuit	223 g	690	47	11	n/l	n/a

BRAND NAME	PRODUCT NAME	SERVING SIZE	CALORIES PER SERVING	TOTAL FAT (G) PER SERVING	SATURATED FAT (G) PER SERVING	TRANS FAT (G) PER SERVING	SAT + TRANS (G)
	Bacon, Egg & Cheese Biscuit	174 g	560	38	11	n/l	n/a
	Ham, Egg & Cheese Biscuit	220 g	560	35	10	n/l	n/a
	Loaded Omelet Biscuit	198 g	640	44	14	n/l	n/a
	Biscuits 'N' Gravy	251 g	530	34	8	n/l	n/a
	Sunrise Croissant with Ham	164 g	430	26	10	n/l	n/a
	Sunrise Croissant with Bacon	138 g	450	29	12	n/l	n/a
	Sunrise Croissant with Sausage	161 g	550	38	15	n/l	n/a
	Sunrise Croissant	57 g	210	10	4	n/l	n/a
	Frisco Breakfast Sandwich	181 g	410	17	7	n/l	n/a
	Tortilla Scrambler	66 g	230	13	6	n/l	n/a
	Loaded Omelet	89 g	270	21	9	n/l	n/a
	Loaded Biscuit 'N' Gravy Breakfast Bowl	326 g	770	54	14	n/l	n/a
	Low Carb Breakfast Bowl	208 g	620	50	21	n/l	n/a
	Pancake Platter	135 g	300	5	1	n/l	n/a
	Big Country Breakfast Platter with Country Ham	377 g	970	53	12	n/l	n/a
	Big Country Breakfast Platter with Bacon	355 g	980	56	13	n/l	n/a
	Big Country Breakfast Platter with Sausage	374 g	1060	64	15	n/l	n/a
	Big Country Breakfast Platter with Chicken	458 g	1140	61	13	n/l	n/a
	Big Country Breakfast Platter with Breaded Pork Chop	455 g	1220	68	13	n/l	n/a
	Big Country Breakfast Platter with Grilled Pork Chop	440 g	1130	61	15	n/l	n/a
	Big Country Breakfast Platter with Country Steak	412 g	1150	68	16	n/l	n/a
	Hash Rounds, small	83 g	260	16	4	n/l	n/a
	Hash Rounds, medium	114 g	350	22	5	n/l	n/a

Hash Rounds, large	151 g	460	29	6	n/l	n/a
American Cheese slice, small	12 g	50	4	3	n/l	n/a
Swiss Cheese slice	16 g	50	4	3	n/l	n/a
Breakfast Ham slice	56 g	60	3	1	n/l	n/a
Country Ham slice	35 g	60	3	2	n/l	n/a
Bacon	2 strips	45	4	1	n/l	n/a
Sausage Patty	33 g	150	14	5	n/l	n/a
Chicken Fillet	117 g	230	11	2	n/l	n/a
Country Steak	71 g	240	18	5	n/l	n/a
Cinnamon 'N' Raisin Biscuit	77 g	280	12	3	n/l	n/a
Lunch and Dinner						
⅓ lb Thickburger	342 g	850	57	22	n/l	n/a
⅓ lb Cheeseburger	254 g	680	39	19	n/l	n/a
⅓ lb Mushroom 'N' Swiss Thickburger	276 g	720	42	21	n/l	n/a
⅓ lb Bacon Cheese Thickburger	333 g	910	63	24	n/l	n/a
⅓ lb Low Carb Thickburger	245 g	420	32	12	n/l	n/a
½ lb Six Dollar Burger	412 g	1060	72	30	n/l	n/a
½ lb Grilled Sourdough Thickburger	382 g	1020	73	30	n/l	n/a
⅔ lb Double Thickburger	471 g	1240	90	38	n/l	n/a
⅔ lb Double Bacon Cheese Thickburger	462 g	1300	96	40	n/l	n/a
⅔ lb Monster Thickburger	413 g	1410	107	45	n/l	n/a
Charbroiled Chicken Club Sandwich	277 g	560	30	8	n/l	n/a
Charbroiled BBQ Chicken Sandwich	272 g	415	5	1	n/l	n/a
Big Chicken Fillet Sandwich	362 g	770	36	8	n/l	n/a
Spicy Chicken Sandwich	160 g	470	26	5	n/l	n/a
Regular Roast Beef	137 g	330	16	7	n/l	n/a
Big Roast Beef	199 g	470	23	10	n/l	n/a
Hot Ham 'N' Cheese	191 g	420	18	10	n/l	n/a

BRAND NAME	PRODUCT NAME	SERVING SIZE	CALORIES PER SERVING	TOTAL FAT (G) PER SERVING	SATURATED FAT (G) PER SERVING	TRANS FAT (G) PER SERVING	SAT + TRANS (G)
	Big Hot Ham 'N' Cheese	244 g	520	24	13	n/l	n/a
	Hot Dog	152 g	420	30	12	n/l	n/a
	Slammers	95 g	240	12	5	n/l	n/a
	Slammers with Cheese	108 g	280	16	8	n/l	n/a
	3-Piece Chicken Strips	145 g	380	21	4	n/l	n/a
	5-Piece Chicken Strips	241 g	630	34	6	n/l	n/a
	Kid's Meal, 2 Chicken Strips	175 g	500	25	5	n/l	n/a
	Kid's Meal, 2 Slammers	270 g	720	35	13	n/l	n/a
Sides							
	Grilled Onions	28 g	35	3	3	n/l	n/a
	Bacon	1½ strips	60	5	2	n/l	n/a
	American Cheese Slice, large	16 g	60	5	4	n/l	n/a
	Swiss Cheese Slice	16 g	50	4	3	n/l	n/a
	Au Jus Sauce	85 g	10	0	0	n/l	n/a
	Fried Chicken Breast	148 g	370	15	4	n/l	n/a
	Fried Chicken Wing	66 g	200	8	2	n/l	n/a
	Fried Chicken Thigh	121 g	330	15	4	n/l	n/a
	Fried Chicken Leg	69 g	170	7	2	n/l	n/a
	French Fries, Kid's	79 g	250	12	3	n/l	n/a
	French Fries, small	126 g	390	19	4	n/l	n/a
	French Fries, medium	166 g	520	24	5	n/l	n/a
	French Fries, large	193 g	610	28	6	n/l	n/a
	Crispy Curls, small	109 g	340	17	4	n/l	n/a
	Crispy Curls, medium	132 g	410	20	5	n/l	n/a
	Crispy Curls, large	153 g	480	23	6	n/l	n/a

Item						
Cole Slaw, small—1 serving	113 g	170	10	2	n/l	n/a
Cole Slaw, large—3 servings	113 g	170	10	2	n/l	n/a
Mashed Potatoes, small—1 serving	142 g	90	2	0	n/l	n/a
Mashed Potatoes, large—3 servings	142 g	90	2	0	n/l	n/a
Chicken Gravy	43 g	20	1	0	n/l	n/a
Honey Mustard Dipping Sauce	28 g	110	9	1.5	n/l	n/a
Ranch Dressing Dipping Sauce	28 g	160	16	3	n/l	n/a
BBQ Sauce Dipping Sauce	14 g	15	0	0	n/l	n/a
Sweet N Sour Dipping Sauce	28 g	45	0	0	n/l	n/a
Mayonnaise (packet)	12 g	90	9	1.5	n/l	n/a
Hot Sauce (packet)	7 g	0	0	0	n/l	n/a
Horseradish Sauce (packet)	7 g	25	2	0	n/l	n/a
Ketchup (packet)	9 g	10	0	0	n/l	n/a

Desserts

Item						
Chocolate Chip Cookie	68 g	290	11	5	n/l	n/a
Apple Turnover	85 g	290	15	5	n/l	n/a
Hand-Dipped Ice Cream, single	n/l	n/l	n/l	n/l	n/l	n/a
Hand-Dipped Ice Cream, double	n/l	n/l	n/l	n/l	n/l	n/a

Acknowledgments

I am indebted to many people for helping to bring this book to life. Many thanks to Lindsey Moore, assistant editor at Three Rivers Press, and Kathryn McHugh, former associate editor at Three Rivers Press, who guided this book from concept to reality; to Mary Ann Naples at The Creative Culture; to my husband, Michael Hobbs, who assisted with research and editing; and to Kristen Beam and Daniel Beavers, who helped compile nutrient data. I am grateful to all.

Index

Page numbers in *italic* refer to references in Food Guide and Fat Gram Counter

Recipe Credits

About the Author

SUZANNE HAVALA HOBBS is a registered, licensed dietitian and a nationally recognized writer on food, nutrition, and health policy. She holds a doctorate in health policy and administration from the University of North Carolina at Chapel Hill, where she is a clinical assistant professor in the School of Public Health and director of the doctoral program in health leadership.

She has written ten books, including *Being Vegetarian for Dummies*, *Vegetarian Cooking for Dummies*, *The Natural Kitchen*, and *Good Foods, Bad Foods: What's Left to Eat?* She is a contributing writer for *Bottom Line/Personal* and *Vegetarian Times*, and is a nutrition editor for *Vegetarian Journal*.

Through her newspaper column, "On the Table," Suzanne explores topics related to food, nutrition, and food-related policy issues. The column appears weekly in the *News & Observer* of Raleigh, North Carolina, and the *Charlotte Observer*. An archive of "On the Table" columns can be found at www.onthetable.net.

Suzanne's advice has been quoted in the *New York Times*, *Parade*, *SELF Magazine*, *Shape*, *Vegetarian Times*, *Runner's World*, *New Woman*, *YM*, *Omni*, *Sassy*, and *Harper's Bazaar* and in appearances on *Good Morning America*, *Weekend Today in New York*, and *The Susan Powter Show*.

Suzanne is a member of the American Public Health Association, American Dietetic Association, National Association of Science Writers, American Society of Journalists and Authors, and Association of Food Journalists. She serves on the board of directors of the Association of Health Care Journalists and the Center for Excellence in Health Care Journalism, and is a member of the board of trustees of the North Carolina Writers Network.

She lives in Chapel Hill, North Carolina.